Lifesaving and Marine Safety

COMPANION TITLES FROM NEW CENTURY

The New Science of Skin and Scuba Diving

The New Science of Skin and Scuba Diving Workbook

First Aid for Boaters and Divers

Getting in Shape for Skin & Scuba Diving

Lifesaving and Marine Safety

UNITED STATES LIFESAVING ASSOCIATION

Association Press
NEW CENTURY PUBLISHERS, INC.

Printing Code
11   12   13   14   15   16

Librar of Congress Cataloging in Publication Data
Main entry under title:

Lifesaving and marine safety.

   Includes index.
   1. Lifeguards—Training of. 2. Lifesaving—
Study and teaching. I. D'Arnall, Douglas G.
II. United States Lifesaving Association.
GV838.74.L53   363.1'4   81-11134
ISBN 0-8329-0113-X   AACR2

Contents

Foreword

HISTORY OF LIFESAVING IN THE UNITED STATES

The first recorded occurrence of lifesaving was inaugurated by the Chinese to protect lives on their major rivers prior to the establishment in the Occident in Europe. Other pioneer lifesaving efforts were established in the 17th and 18th centuries by the French, Dutch and Commonwealth countries. The founding of the Massachussetts Humane Society in 1785 commenced the history of lifesaving in America. Lifeguards were all volunteers and the Society presented medals and small cash emoluments to individuals who frequently made dramatic rescues in adverse conditions.

In 1878, under the guidance of Sumner I. Kimball, the chief of the Revenue Cutter Service, the Secretary of the Treasury created a separate bureau named the United States Lifesaving Service, which merged with the Revenue Cutter Service in 1915 to create the United States Coast Guard. During its short life, the United States Lifesaving Service was credited with saving 175,000 lives.

The first official lifeguard on the Pacific coast, George Douglas Freeth, was the son of a Hawaiian princess and American father. Freeth developed an early lifeguard training program at Redondo Beach, California and was awarded the gold medal of the United States Lifesaving Service for the rescue of seven fishermen whose boats were being smashed against the Venice Beach Breakwater on December 8, 1908. Freeth is also credited with introducing the sport of surfing to the mainland.

In the first decade of the twentieth century Americans on both ocean coasts, the Gulf of Mexico, and throughout the Territory of Hawaii discovered the joys of a beach outing during their increased leisure time. The only paid lifeguards were those working the large hotels. Rescue equipment provided at public beaches was limited and usually consisted of a line and floatation devices. In Venice Beach, California, at the suggestion of George Freeth, brass ship's bells were mounted on posts so that anyone spotting a distressed swimmer could ring the bell to signal for help.

The first rescue float was developed in 1897 by Captain Harry Sheffield for a lifesaving club in South Africa. It was four feet long, sharply pointed at both ends and quite heavy. The design was soon modified in the United States and the heavy sheet metal was replaced with copper, then aluminum. An inflatable rescue tube that could be snapped around the waist of a victim was developed in the 1930s. When the famous Duke Paoa Kanhanamoku, father of Hawaiian surfing, visited the west coast in 1913, he introduced his redwood surfboard to the Long Beach, California lifeguards. Shortly thereafter the paddleboard became an important rescue tool to lifeguards everywhere.

The growth of lifeguards in America was not orderly. It took 13 drownings in a flash rip current in 1918 for the city of San Diego, California to see a need for an organized service. The city of Long Beach, California hired its first municipal guard, Hinnie Zimmerman, in 1908. In 1918 the city of Huntington Beach, California hired two part-time lifeguards, Henry Brouhs and Robert Nut. The city of Los Angeles began its lifeguard service in 1925 and their soon-to-be-chief, Myron Cox, was the first to express the concept "Prevent a rescue instead of making one," which is still the basic philosophy of lifeguarding today.

Lifeguard history abounds with names of great athletes and lifesaving pioneers: Herb Barthels (holder of the world five-mile swim record in 1932); Wally O'Connor (three-time Olympic medal winner); Thomas E. Blake (champion surfer and inventor of the paddleboard); Preston "Pete" Peterson, famous tandem surfer and superb boatman; Dutch Miller, who, with his brother Vic, guided Long Beach's Lifeguard Service for over half a century; and Frank "Bud" Stevenson, whose 40-year career with Los Angeles County lifeguards began in 1930.

These pioneers of lifeguarding and the hundreds of other dedicated lifeguards who were there on both coasts when it all began have left a heritage of which lifeguards today can be justifiably proud.

UNITED STATES LIFESAVING ASSOCIATION

The USLA was conceived in 1964 and incorporated in the State of California as a nonprofit educational and charitable organization in

1966 under the name "National Surf Life Saving Association of America" (NSLSA). In 1979 the NSLSA expanded its membership to include all open water and surf lifeguards and changed its name to properly reflect the scope of its membership.

The primary purpose of the USLA is to better aquaint the public, through educational means, in all areas of aquatic safety. Concurrent with this purpose, the USLA promotes and develops the highest level of surf and open water lifesaving methods and techniques and familiarizes the general public with the functions and services of the marine safety and lifeguard services in their community. In pursuance of these goals, the USLA makes available to schools, civic groups, and other individuals and organizations various educational films, manuals, and texts.

The USLA is nationally recognized as the most authoritative body in the field of open water surf lifeguarding and marine safety. The USLA is affiliated internationally with the World Life Saving Association and conducts international educational exchange programs as a further means to achieve its humanitarian goals.

1

The Role of the Professional Lifeguard

When Commodore Wilbert E. Longfellow initiated the Life Saving Service of the American National Red Cross in 1914, he coined the slogan, "Everyone a swimmer, every swimmer a lifesaver," which reflects the sound philosophy that for the individual, the best kind of lifesaving is being able to swim well. However, even able swimmers can find themselves in aquatic difficulty. This reality underlines the primary responsibility of the professional lifeguard—to protect the lives of individuals not only swimming or bathing but also engaging in other water recreations.

Beyond this fundamental calling of the lifeguard, in order that agency and community needs are met fully, lifeguards must often become proficient in additional areas of marine safety and law enforcement. The scope of responsibility varies from the tower guard with the sole obligation of protecting persons in his assigned area, to the year-round professional, often both deputized as a special police officer and trained fully in fire suppression.

The Code of Ethics of the United States Lifesaving Association establishes for all lifeguards a remarkable commitment:

The United States Lifesaving Association, realizing the fundamental responsibilities of a professional lifeguard toward mankind, the trust and

1

confidence placed in him, the unwavering devotion to duty required of him and the dignity commensurate with his position, recognizes ethical principles.

The member will:

Serve mankind through the diligent protection of life and property.

Remain totally loyal to his employer, community, state and nation.

Promote through youth and adult groups understanding of the privileges and responsibilities of American Democracy.

Fulfill his responsibility by honoring, dignifying and actively supporting his profession.

Recognize the value of the profession and promote its future by inspiring promising young people to prepare for it.

Recognize the responsibility of the professional group for the conduct of its members.

Maintain relationships with associates based on mutual integrity, understanding and respect.

Maintain his health and high level of physical fitness.

Attempt to think clearly and maintain objective points of view on controversial questions, being ever mindful of the welfare of others.

Show that he has a position of special trust and adhere to the standard of personal conduct acceptable for professional standing in the community.

Understand the requirements of effective organization and willingly work through channels.

Never allow personal feelings or danger to self to deter him from his responsibilities.

The member will strive to achieve these objectives and ideals, dedicating himself before God to his chosen profession.

This code of conduct clearly indicates the caliber of the profession. A professional lifeguard is a multifaceted individual who should have a thorough knowledge of some or all of the following marine-safety-oriented subjects—methods of effecting all forms of swimming rescues; resuscitation and paramedical first aid; vessel and aircraft rescues; effects of marine environment; search and recovery techniques including scuba (self-contained underwater breathing apparatus); operation and maintenance of power rescue boats and rescue vehicles including all equipment thereon; methods of effecting cliff rescues; evacuation of flood victims; prevention of accidents; coordination of activities with other emergency agencies in the local vicinity such as fire, police, ambulance services, U. S. Coast Guard; operation of multichanneled radios and telephone switchboards; and elements of supervision and administration.

In addition to subjects directly related to safety and lifesaving, the professional should have a working knowledge of other correlated duties, including all phases of swimming instruction; operation of junior lifeguard programs; lectures to community interest groups on water safety, first aid, and other related marine safety subjects; and instruction for classes in aquatic safety at local elementary schools, secondary schools, and colleges. These subjects can be multiplied in direct relation to the commitment to community involvement.

Unlike other public safety personnel, lifeguards are not primarily on call during or after distress situations develop, but rather must have the unique capability of recognizing potential dangers before they occur. The old maxim, "An ounce of prevention is worth a pound of cure," is fully applicable to lifeguarding. The visual and instinctive reaction to signs of trouble are the real keys to prevention: To wait until called would possibly never prevent a drowning. In this regard the proficient professional adheres to four basic principles:

1. Prevent all possible emergencies by recognizing danger signs.
2. Exercise good judgment as to the priority of the emergencies.
3. Know how to effect a rescue in the quickest, most efficient manner.
4. Know what to do with the victim upon returning to shore.

Experience has demonstrated that the intelligent application of these four principles will serve to significantly guarantee the safe operation of any aquatic recreational area.

While the employment of many lifeguards is seasonal, many locales have a climate and year-round influx of visitors that necessitate full-time professional lifeguards. In most instances, these professionals are supplemented by part-time lifeguards during peak periods—summer, heavy surf days, warm off-season periods, holidays, special events, and other times when the public safety mandates them. These part-time guards should meet the same standards as the full-time professionals.

The recurrent part-time lifeguard should be employed on the basis of several important factors. Of primary consideration should be individual aptitude, personal qualifications, experience, and past performance. Since it is mandatory for the administrator to provide the best possible protection for each dollar spent but simultaneously to make the selection process as objective as possible, a policy for selecting recurrent lifeguards provides substantial guidance.

Because of their overall contribution to the safety of the communities they serve, most professional lifeguards are paid as well as other public safety officers such as police or firemen. Recurrent lifeguards are paid on many different scales—some hourly, some daily, some weekly. In places where year-round professional staffs are maintained, lifeguards are paid additional increments; and salaries reflect their added responsibilities as rescue vehicle operators, scuba team members, and temporary or full-time supervisory personnel. The rate of pay is determined by the agency providing the lifeguard service and adjusted on the basis of additional responsibilities.

In most instances, the basic professional lifeguard schedule is a forty-hour, five-day week. However, some lifeguards may be scheduled on a ten-hour, four-day week in order to provide increased coverage for the public during the critical early morning and late afternoon hours. During peak beach usage, scheduling may have to be further altered to guarantee that maximum protection and coverage are provided. Compensation for these extra working hours can be paid in a variety of ways. Two common methods are to grant time off during slack periods for overtime work during peak periods or to pay overtime on either a straight time or a time and a half basis.

Whenever possible, work schedules should be made up and posted well in advance. Normal rest breaks for workouts and lunches should also be recorded on the schedule and religiously followed. A lifeguard who cannot work an assigned shift should notify the supervisor without delay so a viable replacement can be made. The lifeguard should arrive sufficiently in advance of the scheduled work period to report in, be inspected by the supervisor, and be on station at the time scheduled. If appropriate or expected breaks are not scheduled in writing, proper authorization should be obtained prior to leaving an assigned post.

In any well-administered marine safety agency, each lifeguard should be aware of his or her position within the organization. Organizational charts should be readily available, and this important information should be included in an agency or departmental operations manual available to all employees. It serves to clarify positions, pinpoint responsibility, and build an esprit de corps vital to the fully functioning marine safety mission.

Lifeguard uniforms are also important. An individual lifeguard should be readily distinguishable from the patrons surrounding his assigned post. When a patron needs assistance, in almost all instances there is little time. The lifeguard who is on station in appropriate attire will be easily located without delay. There is also the "public relations" aspect of the uniform: No other member of the agency is as closely observed by so many people as the lifeguard on duty.

The appearance of the lifeguard while on a duty has a direct correlation with public confidence; his ability to perform his duties proficiently. The positive image of the lifeguard should be maintained without exception. Further, experience shows that general beach problems, many which do not relate directly to the water environment, are more readily, easily, and efficiently solved by neat, uniformed, clean-appearing personnel. Detailed suggested uniform regulations and requirements are discussed at length in Chapter 10.

SUGGESTED PREREQUISITES FOR LIFEGUARD TRAINING

All marine safety agencies establish minimum requirements for admittance into their lifeguard-training programs. Prerequisites vary from agency to agency, city to city, state to state, and nation to nation. Suggested prerequisites follow:

1. Age seventeen
2. Physical examination
   a. normal hearing;
   b. 20–20 uncorrected vision;
   c. normal heart, lungs, and reflexes;
   d. no disabling deformities or conditions; and
   e. demonstration of ability to handle any and all situations indigenous to area of responsibility
3. Practical tests
   a. 1000-meter swim in sixteen minutes; or
   b. 500-meter swim in seven and a half minutes; and/or
   c. 1200-meter run-swim-run.

By its intrinsic nature, lifeguarding places extreme limits on the physical and mental alertness of its personnel. The entire human mechanism is fully involved in its duties and demands. Maximum effort is the rule and not the exception. To achieve this maximum performance, the individual lifeguard must develop and maintain strong positive attitudes toward personal health and fitness and participate in continuing physical and mental in-service training.

The marine safety agency has a vested and justifiable interest in the personal health habits of its personnel because they can and do affect the performance of the employee and particularly of the lifeguard. The agency objective is the development of health standards that eliminate as many negative influences as possible in order to achieve the end goal of maximized mental and physical fitness. In the interest of alertness, alcohol and drugs are two prime negative influences deleterious to full performance that professionals should avoid. Under no circumstance should use of alcohol or drugs be tolerated prior to or during working hours. Pernicious drug abuse should receive the constant attention of supervisorial and managerial personnel. In the interest of public safety, no known drug user or alcoholic should remain on staff. Current research indicates that tobacco smoking is also detrimental to optimal fitness, and policy on tobacco should be periodically reviewed.

All lifeguards experience the rigorous exposure to the natural elements inherent in the job. Overexposure to the sun can be avoided by limiting the first initial exposure, by utilizing sunshades and the protection of a lifeguard tower, by wearing appropriate

uniform clothing, and/or by using a suntan lotion containing ultra-
violet ray protective chemicals. A good pair of dark sunglasses is
highly recommended. Protection against sunless cold, damp
weather is equally important. Every lifeguard must have warm,
loose, rain resistant, easy to shed clothing mandated as part of his
required uniform. Footwear designed for warmth and safety is
important as well. The properly clothed lifeguard functions fully.

Personal health should be of primary concern in everything a
lifeguard does in fulfilling the functions of his duties. For both
health and sanitary reasons, cleanliness of personal self and of on-
duty and off-duty apparel is an absolute necessity. The personal
appearance of each and every lifeguard reflects the alertness, pride,
and professional attitudes of every other guard in the service. The
lifeguard must always respect the importance of his public image.
While identified as a lifeguard either on or off duty, his responsibility to safety carries with it a public attentiveness to all
situations in which he involves himself. Horseplay or stunts that
may result in personal injury display an inappropriate disregard for
safety, public or private, and a lack of maturity that serves as a poor
example to the viewing public.

Many professional lifeguards follow a regimen of proper nutrition,
adequate rest, and adherence to a continuing physical fitness
program to assure their maximal physical and mental conditioning.
Such positive attention to personal well-being also assures the
ability to recuperate rapidly from periods of full exertion or from
cuts and other wounds often caused by the aquatic environment.
Working in a damp atmosphere is often conducive to infection, so
wounds should receive immediate and proper treatment.

IN-SERVICE TRAINING

Since the lifeguard must maintain a high degree of physical and
mental readiness, comprehensive training programs for both full-
time and part-time lifeguards are imperative. The curriculum in
these agency training sessions should be well thought out and well
rounded, to include all of the following—physical training, classroom instruction, skills development, public relations, and specific
programmatic features designed to instill professional attitudes
toward lifeguarding. Whenever appropriate, group training sessions
are an excellent tool for establishing and maintaining the much-
desired esprit de corps in and between all members of the marine
safety force. Time alloted each curricular phase of the training
program should be dictated by the various problems that arise under
actual agency working conditions and experiences. In this fashion,

each agency training program is uniquely tailored to meet the real requirements of the agency it serves.

An aspect of training common to all types of lifeguarding, indoors or outdoors, is, of course, swimming, During the peak season, all lifeguards should swim a minimum of 400 yards daily and a minimum of 1000 yards on a weekly basis in the very environment in which they work and must function. There is no substitute for running: Running is a necessity for all ocean lifeguards. A daily run of a mile, prior to or immediately after the swimming workout, is adequate. During the off season, a once weekly timed performance swim test should insure a proper level of fitness. Workouts on rescue surfboats or paddleboards as well as with rescue rowboats or dories may be an integral, supplemental, or optional part of any overall program.

Marine safety agencies requiring proficiency in scuba techniques should require their divers to practice dive once weekly for physiological, psychological, and safety reasons. Workout schedules, whenever possible, should be organized and posted in advance, but at no time should they be allowed to interfere with or jeopardize the safety and well-being of the public.

Beyond the fundamentals of lifeguarding, which need constant reinforcement, the classroom instruction portion of the total training program should reflect the specific commitments of the marine agency to their particular public. One of the primary objectives in this phase of the training is the constant review and upgrading of techniques (1) specific to the particular agency and (2) pertinent to agency community responsibilities. Subject matter therefore will vary, but in the consideration of curriculum selection, the following topics are deserving of serious consideration for inclusion—(1) modern techniques in effecting water rescues, (2) latest methods of resuscitation, and (3) up-to-date first aid techniques and emergency care.

Agency personnel responsible for the implementation of the training program should make liberal use of the various authorities available from within the community they serve. Medical doctors, lawyers, police officers, firemen, and other such individuals are usually eager to help and pleased to be asked. The community public service organizations, such as the local chapter of the American National Red Cross, the American Heart Association, and others, are readily available resources to complement and supplement intensive training. Audiovisual materials often available from these sources include films, film strips, tapes, and videotapes. Such materials immeasurably enhance the instruction process.

Just as the prospective lawyer pleads his case in moot court, so do mock emergency situations serve to better prepare the lifeguard—professional or recurrent, new or experienced—mentally as well as physically. The maintenance of practical application drills as part of the curriculum should stress all aspects of the training curriculum itself, providing trainee experience that faithfully duplicates actual encounters. For supervisorial personnel, these training drills may further serve as important evaluation tools for assessing the capabilities of the trainees.

The underlying commitment of the entire in-service training program is the inculcation of a professional approach to the lifesaving career. A philosophy of positive attitudes, which reflect personal pride and a dedication to public safety, should be the general thrust of all training. Agency supervisors must understand that a lifeguard not in the best physical and psychological condition, a lifeguard insufficiently skilled in rescue techniques or first aid or any other operational duty, a lifeguard who maintains less than the highest personal standards and attitudes is a lifeguard capable of embarassment to himself, his agency, and his profession and, under extreme possibility, being the direct cause of an unnecessary injury or loss of life.

Intra- and interagency lifeguard competitions are positive fitness, morale, and public relations events. Competing lifeguards and competing agencies are at their best during contests and meets. Both loyalty to the agency and personal pride and confidence are invariably developed and enhanced through competetion. The desire to win instills a further desire to attain optimal efficiency in the use of lifeguard rescue equipment. Nor can the public relations value of competitions by underplayed. In real life, few patrons can or will observe an actual rescue in progress and thereby fully appreciate the physical and mental discipline of the lifeguard, but well-planned competitions offer unique opportunities for the public to view the lifeguard in 100 percent effort. Personnel in charge of the physical layout of contests and meets should carefully plan for spectator visibility. The competitors themselves should wear distinctive caps (aqualids) or uniforms or both, so they stand out. If available, a knowledgeable and experienced announcer can do much not only to add color to the events but to dispense important information to the "captured audience" of interested spectators. Chapter 10 details various recommended events.

PREVENTIVE LIFEGUARDING

The late Duke Paoa Kahanamoku, the swimming star of the 1912 Olympic Games at Stockholm, Sweden, and the father of modern surfing, was a lifeguard for several years at the Beach Club in Santa Monica, California, and believed that the "best lifeguard anticipates and thereby prevents accidents." Preventive lifeguarding is the essence of the lifeguard mission. It is the term applied to a technique that precludes an accident by either eliminating or minimizing a hazard or hazardous behavior. Since accidents in swimming, surfing, or other aquatic recreational areas can result in the most serious consequences—including death—it is imperative that all lifeguards develop maximum skills in preventive lifeguarding.

Many accidents that could have been prevented are caused by natural factors in the aquatic environment—for example, water too shallow for diving or sudden drop-offs that plunge waders into deep water. Compound these with hazardous behavior such as roughhousing or horseplay or an unsafe individual act such as attempting to swim too far underwater and the crucial role of preventive lifeguarding is vividly presented. Patron behavior that might endanger their lives and many others is quickly recognized by the aware lifeguard as an invitation to disaster. If accidents are to be avoided, injuries minimized, and lives saved, preventive lifeguarding must be vigilantly practiced by all agency personnel.

In order to prevent all possible accidents, marine safety agencies train their lifeguards to be alert to the following:

1. Swimming in remote areas. Swimmers should be strongly encouraged to confine their aquatic activity within the limits of guarded areas only.
2. Removal of hazards. When conditions permit, the guard, after reporting to the duty station, should remove from the beach or shore such debris as glass, tin cans, posts, open fires, and any other litter; and should check the surfline for logs and timber and for any other dangerous objects that might cause injury to the public. However, it should be a prime goal of any marine safety agency to relieve the lifeguard of beach cleaning chores. Such cleaning functions should be assigned to maintenance personnel.
3. Dangerous marine life. All beach patrons should be made aware of the presence of dangerous marine life whenever necessary. Injured or sick seals, jellyfish, Portugese men-of-war, stingrays, sea urchins, or sharks are threats to the safety of the beach, and only by alerting all using the facility can safety be assured.
4. Riptides, backwashes, run-outs, lateral and other currents, or heavy surf conditions. Well-trained lifeguards readily recognize these ocean conditions and should direct all patrons away from these problem areas without delay. Warning signs or flags should be posted whenever possible to supplement verbal warnings given by the guards.
5. Swimming, both above and under the water, close to hazardous obstructions. Lifeguards should keep all swimmers and bathers away from obstructions such as piers, pilings, groins, jetties, and other manmade hazards such as artificial reefs. Not only do they often

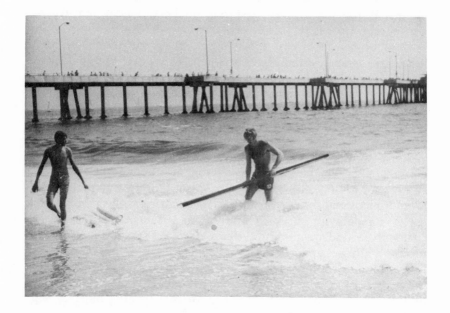

create dangerous currents, but they also often have sharp cutting edges and surfaces.

6. Changing bottom conditions. From time to time, without prior warning, the bottom conditions of a sandy or muddy bottom will change so as to endanger the safety of poor swimmers or nonswimmers. Lifeguards must be on the alert for such changes and keep patrons away from these areas.

7. Swimming too far from shore. Guards should be alert for the swimmer who ventures too far from the shoreline. Swimmers who wish to swim a distance should be encouraged to swim parallel to the shore at a reasonable distance out.

8. Individuals under the influence of alcohol or drugs. Lifeguards must watch for persons who may be under the influence of alcohol or drug intoxication. Any such individual should be removed immediately from the beach.

9. Inflated air mattresses. Patrons who use these devices are in danger of being carried out to sea or dashed on the beach by a breaking wave. A speeding air mattress propelled through the surf by a breaking wave can also inflict serious injuries on others in the water. Both the use and type of these devices should be carefully controlled. Critical neck and back injuries have occurred when inflatable apparatus has been used.

10. Horseplay on the beach. While the primary responsibility of the lifeguard is to protect the patron in the water, he has a further responsibility for the safety of those patrons on the beach. Acts that jeopardize the safety of either the actor and other patrons or both must be discouraged.

11. Surfing areas. Absolutely no swimming should be permitted in areas set aside exclusively for board surfing. A surfboard on the loose is a lethal weapon. Surfers riding incoming waves can run right over swimmers. To permit swimming in surfing areas or surfing in swimming areas is a simple invitation to disaster.
12. Skin and scuba divers. Spear fishing on a swimming beach should be strongly discouraged and, if permitted, strictly regulated and controlled.

All new lifeguards must be instructed in how to guard densely populated beaches with subsequent heavy water activity. The following principles of operation will help serve to establish proper guidelines for overall beach surveillance. First, each lifeguard should establish his perimeter area—that area under his surveillance. This area will include the specific beach under his direct supervision, plus an overlapping territory involving about one-third of the area assigned to the adjacent guards, to create an overlap of surveillance.

Second, any swimmer beyond a reasonable distance offshore should be encouraged to return beachward to a safer distance. At the beginning of each working shift, to ascertain any dangers that may exist in his assigned area, a thorough observational checkout should be made by the lifeguard. He must also be aware of any action of the changing tide that might be hazardous to this area. Finally, throughout his tour of duty, he must be vigilant for any unusual behavior by any individual or group of individuals within his perimeter section.

Since by nature individuals vary not only in physical size and ability but also in knowledge of ocean conditions, it is difficult to determine a specific bather or swimmer danger zone. There is one generalization, however, that does apply: Swimmers who are in chest high or deeper water require more attention than those in shallower water, and children always require the closest scrutiny.

Many experienced lifeguards can spot a potential rescue as the bather enters the water by his appearance and by his actions. A basic tipoff to the condition and ability of a swimmer is his reaction to cold water. Also, the manner in which the bather passes through a wave can be a tipoff. If he turns his back to the surf, the resuce potential increases.

A guard must also be aware of local weather conditions and what effect they will have on the safety of bathers. Danger areas that are rendered even more hazardous by bad weather or dangers created by an increase in wind, surf, or current conditions must be dealt with spontaneously. Under these weather conditions, the two best approaches to guarantee public safety are to (1) assign additional lifeguards to the area or (2) relocate the patrons to a safer area. A system of colored flags or easy to read signs can be employed to warn bathers of water hazards.

Inexperienced lifeguards must be stationed in such a manner that they may be closely supervised by either (1) year-round professionals or (2) veteran recurrent lifeguards. This method of scheduling is an internal preventive measure that achieves two objectives: First, it provides for maximal public safety, and second, it allows for further learning situations for new lifeguards either directed by or observing the veteran.

Preventive lifeguarding is the best lifeguarding, and it will invariably reduce the incidence of actual rescues and of accidents in any specific aquatic area where it is diligently utilized. For this reason, preventive lifeguarding constitutes one of the most valid lifesaving techniques. It must be remembered, however, that there are circumstances when the guard must act instantaneously, as lives can be lost in seconds. The lifeguard must be able to evaluate these situations immediately and react appropriately.

Action takes precedence over prevention.

FIRST AID AND EMERGENCY CARE

For the lifeguard there is no greater responsibility than the first aid treatment and care of injured patrons or victims of sudden illness, whether marine related or not. Lifeguards must be trained to dispense first aid in a quick and efficient manner, specializing in first aid for situations specific to the marine environment. For this reason, lifeguard training officers emphasize sound first aid training and maintain a continuing liaison with medical experts so as to remain abreast of new developments and new, more effective first aid methods.

Marine safety agencies either include first aid training as a prerequisite for employment or include first aid training in their formal training program for new lifeguard candidates. It is imperative that every lifeguard, irregardless of his assignment, have a basic minimum first aid background that includes certification in standard first aid and personal safety and in cardio-pulmonary resuscitation (CPR). It is also strongly recommended that lifeguards receive advanced training in the care and management of head, neck, and back injuries in the aquatic environment.

Those lifeguard personnel who are classified as "full-time" and/or who are assigned to a supervisory position should be certified as EMT-1 so that they can provide competent backup skills and knowledge for major emergencies and assist paramedical personnel, who are frequently called in to assist.

It is also paramount that frequent in-service training sessions in first aid and emergency care be conducted, with emphasis on major skills such as CPR, splinting, bandaging, and transportation. Illnesses and injuries with which lifeguards have infrequent contact should also be periodically reviewed; otherwise, the experience of the lifeguard with these first aid possibilities will become too limited. The sagacious lifeguard agency will also meet periodically with local paramedical, ambulance, and hospital emergency room personnel, so that medical aid incidents can be critiqued and the level of mutual cooperation and service can be constantly improved and upgraded.

Every lifeguard facility should have a complete inventory of first aid supplies. Such an inventory is for usage at the facility itself as well as serving as the supply source for stocking emergency vehicles and individual first aid kits. The variety of supplies stored will vary from area to area, depending on local environment characteristics and the types of accidents and injuries that most frequently occur in the locale. Actual experience in different geographic areas will best determine projected budgeting of supplies.

2

Public Relations

In an address to the Young People's Society, Greenpoint Presbyterian Church, Brooklyn, New York, in 1901, Mark Twain admonished his youthful audience: "Always do right. This will gratify some people and astonish the rest." President Harry S. Truman kept this saying on his desk in the Oval Office. Every lifeguard in his relations with the public he serves must follow its counsel. Any public service agency, and particularly one dealing with safety functions such as lifeguarding, should consider a public relations program as both a necessary and an ongoing service.

An aquatic safety agency public relations program should be geared to meet two basic objectives—first, the creation of reciprocal understanding and good will between the agency and the public it serves, and second, the creation of the conviction in the public at large that the public agency is an "authoritative body" in those areas for which it bears responsibility. Gaining the support, cooperation, and confidence of the public through persuasion is part of the day-by-day work of every public agency. It is not a once a year, once a month, or once a week affair. It is ongoing and continuous if it is to be effective.

The public needs to know that when educated advice and information are needed on aquatic activities, the lifeguard has that expertise and is anxious to share it with them. In pursuit of this relationship, an increasing number of marine safety agencies employ a full-time public relations director and/or staff. The usefulness of public relations is beyond debate, and a positive PR orientation is a requirement for every successful lifeguard and lifesaving administrator.

The first step for a marine safety agency in setting up a public relations program would be to establish a public relations team. Team members should be well trained in the following areas—(1) basic oceanography, rip currents, wave and tidal actions; (2) aquatic activities particular to the geographical area serviced by the agency; (3) environmental and ecological conditions and factors; (4) agency rescue techniques; (5) speaking with poise before both large and small public and private groups; (6) writing press releases and general writing skills; and (7) performing with high proficiency in some special aquatic activity or related area.

It is important that team members be varied in their fields of specialization to avoid a lack of knowledge in any specific area. Inevitably requests for speakers will be for audiences of varying emphasis and skill levels. Obviously, one or two individual staff members cannot be expected to meet all these varying needs. Ideally, it is good to have experts in the areas of cardio-pulmonary resuscitation, diving safety, boating safety, surfing safety, swimming safety, and any other areas of particular importance to the agency locale. Utilizing this system of speaker availability enables the agency to not only reach a wider spectrum of the public it serves, but also to create and sustain a true image of agency expertise.

Both for agencies utilizing staff members to fulfill public relations functions and for those with funds to hire specific staff, the eight major public relations work classifications developed in a vocational guidance survey conducted by the Educational Committee of the Public Relations Society of America are excellent guidelines. These are:

1. Writing (reports, new releases, booklet texts, radio and television copy, speeches, film sequences, trade paper and magazine articles, product information, and technical material);
2. Editing (employee publications, newsletters, shareholder reports, and other management communications directed to both organization personnel and external groups);
3. Placement (contacts with the press, radio, and television, as well as with magazine, Sunday supplement, and trade editors, to enlist their interest in publishing news and features);
4. Promotion (special events, such as press parties, convention exhibits, and special showings; open house, new facility, anniversary celebrations; special day, week, or month observances; contests and award programs; guest relations; institutional movies; visual aids);

5. Speaking (appearances before groups and the planning requisite to finding appropriate platforms; preparation of speeches for others, organization of speakers' bureau, and the delivery of speeches);
6. Production (knowledge of art and layout for development of brochures, booklets, special reports, photographic communications, and house periodicals as required);
7. Programming (the determination of need, definition of goals, and recommended steps in carrying out the project. This is the highest level job in public relations, one requiring maturity in counseling management);
8. Advertising (advertising name and reputation through purchased time or space. Close coordination with advertising departments is maintained, and frequently the advertising-public relations responsibility is a dual one).

These eight points are of major concern on a daily basis to large corporate or organizational public relations staffs. For the marine safety agency, with its public and nonprofit mission, these guidelines apply only infrequently in some instances, but in the main they detail the types of responsibilities a public relations team must be able to meet. Versatility is the necessary virtue in encounters with the public. "Any time more than two Americans meet on the street," Will Rogers said, "one of them is sure to begin looking around for a gavel to call the meeting to order." The well-selected agency public relations staff is ripe, ready, and on its toes, both initiating and awaiting public intercourse.

Once a public relations team has been selected, its first step is to undertake preparation of outlines, visual aids, and safety articles, pursuing the following program:

First, ascertain the variety and scope of projected lectures the agency would wish to make available. Lectures invariably prove to be the most active aspect of a public relations program, and with the passage of time, requests for guest lecturers will progressively increase. They provide the agency with the most flexible medium for presenting its message to the public. Two of the most usual lecture formats are (1) formal lectures before a large or small audience with one speaker or (2) practical factor demonstrations or workshops with one or more lecturers and demonstrators.

The formal lecture, usually presenting an overview of the role of the marine safety agency in the community it serves, in most instances is presented to various groups with a general interest in aquatic safety but on occasion may be requested by a group with a high interest in a specific area of the agency mission. Any member of the PR team can be assigned to deliver a formal lecture, but when the lecture is to be given to a group with a specific interest, a lecturer with full knowledge of that special interest should be assigned.

All formal lectures should include one or all of the following areas of general marine safety interest—local beach conditions and their changes; a basic introduction to ocean currents, including how to spot them and to cope with them; local warning system's, their use and misue; local ordinances pertinent to aquatic activities; basic beach first aid and accident prevention, including CPR; basic lifesaving equipment, rescue techniques, and rescue services available; and what to do in emergencies, how to contact the marine safety agency, its lifeguard services, and other related agencies.

The practical factor demonstrations and workshops are a highly effective method only if limited to small groups; otherwise their effectiveness is greatly diminished. Since they require considerable of time and expertise to set up and operate, they might well be limited to special interest groups such as instructor groups, who in turn can go out and share the knowledge they gain from the practical factor demonstration or workshop.

Subject matter for these important public relations demonstration and workshop sessions is wide ranging and can include any of the following—rescue techniques in the surf, in rip currents, and in other currents and surf conditions; proper exit and entry methods into the surf, on steep sloping beaches, and over rocks and reefs; small boat handling; safety for surfers; and CPR and other specific first aid problems.

Second, prepare by circulating throughout the public relations team a set of basic outlines that set forth the general types of speeches and topics to be offered. A properly prepared outline is not only of great assistance to individual lecturers, but also serves to guarantee that the lecture will follow in logical order and that all speakers will present the same basic information to each group addressed. Outlines should not be so rigid that individual speakers do not feel free to digress when pertinent or to mold their presentation to their audience.

Third, each member of the public relations team should prepare a list of audiovisual aids for the program. Once all suggestions have been considered, obtain, prepare, and organize those audiovisual aids selected for the marine safety PR program. Audiovisual aids are a vital asset when addressing any group of any size. Without them, most audiences will quickly lose interest in the speaker and the subject. Adding sight to sound retains audience interest. As William Werner has pointed out, "Mechanical means of communication have their important places; but they are only adjuncts. None of them can take the place of personal man-to-man contact." As a communication tool for the lecturer, visual and audio aids have become an indispensable adjunct.

These communication tools can include charts, maps, slide series, motion pictures, tapes, demonstration mannequins, displays, and staged events. The gathering together of the selected audiovisual communication aids is the initial step. Methods for obtaining them are suggested as follows:

1. Charts and maps. Charts generally have to be made within the agency itself to depict specific details desired. Maps may be obtainable from other agencies such as the office of the city or county clerk or the automobile clubs, and doctored for agency use. Local Red Cross chapters may also be able to supply some highly usable charts and maps.
2. Slide series. Slides are flexible, which is a distinct advantage over films as they can be moved around or changed to meet the needs of any particular lecture or speaking engagement. Slides may be available from other similar nearby agencies, but in order to provide proper information on local conditions, a marine safety agency will usually have to develop its own slide presentations.
3. Motion pictures. Films on most subjects are usually readily obtainable from other sources. Films on first aid can be obtained from local Red Cross chapters or from local hospitals; on diving safety, from local dive shops and the Department of the Navy; on boating safety films, from the U. S. Coast Guard and from manufacturers of vessels as well; on surfing safety, from the American Surfing Association, the national governing body for amateur surfing in the United States (write the ASA at Box 2622, Newport Beach, California 92663). Films on beach safety are not readily available, and the only source at present is other lifeguard agencies.
4. Tapes. Tapes for specific purposes must be made by the individual agency.
5. Demonstration and training mannequins. Mannequins can be obtained from local Red Cross chapters, local hospitals, and other related agencies.
6. Displays and staged events. Each marine safety agency utilizes its own and available outside resources to mount its own displays and staged events.

Fourth, a pattern of regular releases and public safety articles on topics that your agency wishes to emphasize should be established at the outset. Obtain, or if not obtainable compile and maintain, an up-to-date listing of all local media outlets, including local news agencies, periodicals, radio and television stations, and their various news editors. Methods used by aquatic safety agencies in carrying out these goals include releasing safety articles on various aspects of marine safety before the start of each season and inviting local news media to visit agency facilities to observe rescue techniques and to discuss public safety problems, which often leads to gaining time on local radio and television stations for public safety messages.

Set up a special radio code to alert the media to a major event or resuce (i.e., "Code N" to mean a newsworthy item). The code, given by the first unit on the scene, serves to immediately alert any monitoring media. Special articles on special events and on any major changes in agency activities should be released as a matter of continuing policy. At the end of each year, news releases should be sent to all media outlining what services were rendered to the public, with clear interpretations of why any major increases or decreases of services occurred if they did so occur. In the same year end release, predictions can be included for what the next year may hold in the light of past trends.

Fifth, contact other local public safety agencies with which your agency deals and establish, together with members of their public relations staff or committee, joint training sessions and discussions. By establishing such clear lines of communications, vital links of major importance can be established. Invite the public relations operatives from these agencies to visit the marine safety facilities. With these actions, vital lines of communications are established and clear lines of responsibility are clarified.

Finally, in a complete program to reach the public, the following additional methods of dispensing important information should also be instituted whenever possible:

1. At each station maintained by the agency, a bulletin board should be prominently placed to provide the following information—tides, wind direction and velocity, water/air temperature, water/air visibility, swell size and direction, station hours, personnel, and a daily safety message.
2. Establish, if possible, a telephone with a tape-recorded message to make the information listed in Step 1 immediately available to the public.
3. Maintain a supply of beach directories at each station, and give them out at each public appearance and speaking engagement of an agency staff member.
4. Provide local beach residents with emergency stickers made to fit directly onto the telephone dial carrying lifeguard, police, and fire emergency numbers.
5. Provide divers and dive shops with stickers to place on their equipment and/or their vehicles listing lifeguard, Coast Guard, and recompression chamber telephone numbers.

All six points are vital to the establishment and continuance of a marine safety agency public relations operation. When steps 1 through 4 have been implemented, the new public relations team is ready to begin its public services. Part of any good program is a periodic plan to review every step. Steps 5 and 6 are ongoing; once they have been established, they will tend to take care of themselves, but they also must be subject to periodic review to maintain their effectiveness and to keep current with the constantly changing needs of the public.

Once a public relations program is underway, word of mouth rapidly moves it along in smaller communities, but as a matter of policy, the public relations staff should actively seek contact with various local organizations, including public and private elementary and secondary schools and colleges. The various public and private school systems provide the largest possible exposure and reach the majority of the population with which the agency usually deals directly. Many secondary schools, community colleges, and four-year institutions of higher learning also have diving, boating, and swimming clubs and/or teams that from time to time will request services on specific topics.

Local retailers operating dive shops, surfing shops, and aquatic sports shops are all groups with which contact should be established. Aquatic groups at the YMCA, YWCA, YMHA, and YWHA; American Red Cross chapter groups, local military base service groups; and any other local special interest groups with an emphasis in aquatic activities are also outlets for the dissemination of marine safety information.

To be properly coordinated, it is de rigueur that the public relations team clear all its activities with its administrative body. Speaking engagements should be scheduled during regular agency working hours in order not to upset the agency budget. A speakers bureau should be established, the head of which would work with the individual department heads, to act as a clearinghouse for all requests for speakers from the public relations team. Requests for speakers should be made in writing, and a form should be established for that purpose. A member of the PR team assigned to the speakers bureau should be assigned to keep a log of all speeches given and to tabulate the number of people in each audience.

The speakers bureau is a preplanned means for providing speakers for all groups herein listed and also for service club luncheons; for Chamber of Commerce meetings; and for visiting marine safety personnel from other communities, states, or nations. If the agency has outside legal counsel or other friendly associates, they may also wish to make themselves available for some speaking assignments, especially when requests are made for their special expertise by outside groups. The public relations team should also collect appropriate materials and set up a library by subject matter of topics which lecturers for the speakers bureau will be concerned.

The individual staff member of any marine safety agency most important to any public relations program is the lifeguard in the field. He or she must practice preferred public relations at all times. Because of the nature of his job assignment, the lifeguard has more contact with and is seen by more people than any other member of the agency staff. It is therefore essential that the individual lifeguard conduct himself in a manner that fosters the greatest harmony with the public and reflects only credit upon the agency he serves and represents.

Following are twenty-seven specific and equally important points for a code of conduct for lifeguards. Their adherence to this code will be of inestimable assistance to the efficacy of any agency public relations program. In dealings with the public, whether swimmers, surfers, divers, sunbathers, and others who use the beach for recreation, these twenty-seven guidelines are practicable concepts.

1. An alert, clean-shaven, well-groomed, physically fit lifeguard in proper uniform attire immediately conveys a feeling of security to the public, particularly to parents.
2. The wearing of lifeguard uniforms while off duty should be forbidden, and persons who are not assigned lifeguard duties should not be allowed to wear a regulation lifeguard uniform or parts therefrom. Negative public relations incidents may develop where the public may gain the impression that tax money is supporting persons doing other than their assigned work.
3. Lifeguard stations are offices and must be treated as such. The public should not be permitted to use them as dressing rooms, checkrooms, or club rooms. No one should be permitted in the observation towers except authorized personnel.
4. Lifeguards should not take to or keep in the lifeguard stations, and especially observations towers, anything that will distract or give the appearance of distraction from their assigned duties. Such articles would include musical instruments, unrelated reading materials, photographs, games, television sets, radios, phonographs, or miscellaneous toys.
5. While serving on duty, lifeguards should not participate in beach or water games except in authorized, organized agency workouts that are obviously such to the viewing public.
6. Lifeguard stations and equipment should be maintained in a neat and clean condition at all times. Vehicles should be regularly polished. Assigned lockers should also be neat, clean, and dry. Emergency equipment should always be in ready condition and located in an obvious and highly visible place. Unnecessary noise in and around the stations should be eliminated whenever possible and minimized at all times.

7. The beach should be periodically checked for general cleanliness and for any dangerous conditions such as logs, broken glass, tin cans, or any other items capable of inflicting injury on beach users. If a dangerous, unclean, or unsanitary condition cannot be easily rectified, an immediate report of the situation should be made through appropriate channels.

8. Lifeguards should always be and look alert. They must avoid at all times a slovenly attitude of either mind or body. During working hours, they must understand that it is not professional to lie or sit leisurely on the beach.

9. Lifeguards must never congregate in one location while on duty in such a manner that it appears to the public as if they are engaged in idle chatter. To appear as if a "bull session" is in progress during working hours inevitably conveys the impression that no one is doing his or her job.

10. Lifeguards on duty should avoid any unnecessary familiarity with beach patrons, friends, or relatives while on duty. Such activity and involvement must necessarily detract from required alertness and again conveys to the viewing public the impression of laxity while on duty. If the lifeguard must talk to someone, he should stand at all times facing the water and should allow no one to obstruct his view of the water. All conversation should be both polite and brief.

11. In the use of binoculars, lifeguards should not view objects or persons that do not relate to their duties.

12. No one but authorized personnel should be allowed to use lifeguard equipment as the viewing public assumes that individuals using such equipment are lifeguards, and improper usage serves to discredit the lifeguard service.

13. When addressed, lifeguards should give courteous attention to the public, answering all questions, and when asked a question to which they cannot supply the answer, should direct the person to a source where the information might be available.

14. On a daily basis, all lifeguards should be prepared to supply the public with the following information—air/water temperatures, times of low and high tides, surfing conditions, swimming conditions, skin and scuba diving conditions, or other related water activity conditions in the area of their agency responsibility. All stations posting tide and temperature charts should make sure they are updated daily.

15. Lifeguards must investigate any reasonable public complaint, carefully note any report, and respond to all demands without delay, following agency-mandated courses of action.

16. Lifeguards must understand that their relations with members of the media are crucial to the success of the mission of the marine safety agency they serve. Tactless, conflicting, or carelessly worded statements to the media can be misinterpreted by the public. Off the cuff statements can undo with one stroke all the good work done by the entire agency staff in the field of public relations. At a time of disaster, unusual circumstances, or other newsworthy events, lifeguards are subjected to increased job stress by media reporters or other investigative individuals. The loss of life and/or destruction of public or private property inevitably will involve questions from insurance adjustors, and lifeguards must be careful not to provide

information that is not strictly factual and must avoid all statements based on emotion, supposition, and personal feeling. Statements and comments not based on strict fact may have serious repercussions should civil or criminal lawsuits later arise. In the case of death or serious injury, lifeguards must withhold names and addresses of the victims until their nearest of kin are properly notified. A lifeguard in doubt as to the proper action should immediately refer the news media to his immediate superior or, as in many marine safety agencies, direct all news media requests to the single supervisory officer delegated the responsibility.

17. When in the presence of the public or other employees, lifeguards should address all lifeguard officers by their appropriate titles and not by their first names or nicknames. Lifeguard must always treat supervisorial personnel with the respect due their rank.

18. Lifeguards should treat as confidential official business and activities of the marine safety agency that have not been specifically cleared for release to the public or the media. Lifeguards should not publicly criticize official actions of their agency.

19. Lifeguards must never enter a dispute among themselves in public. At any time, this lowers considerably the confidence of the public in their ability to fulfill their lifesaving mission and during emergency operations is doubly detrimental.

20. Lifeguards using public address systems, telephones, or other means of broadcast or telecast communications must be courteous at all times, liberally using "thank yous" and "pleases" where appropriate.

21. Lifeguards must use the public address (PA) system with discretion. Except in real emergencies, the public should be directed rather than commanded. It should not be necessary to alarm an entire beach area by using the public address system when directing one person. The system should be used only when conditions warrant. Unnecessary usage of the system will disturb many beach patrons to the point where they will register complaints.

22. Lifeguards must never reprimand an individual they have just rescued. They have already learned their lesson. They will know in the future to heed warning signs or obey oral warnings. If a lifeguard feels he wishes to say something, perhaps to a small child, it must be done diplomatically, and a scene must be avoided at all costs.

23. As a matter of policy, if a lifeguard is asked to pose for agency publicity photographs, he should not be asked to pose for any pictures that portray him or her doing anything other than their prescribed responsibilities.

24. Lifeguards must enforce all rules and regulations with tact and diplomacy, particularly under emergency or stress conditions. If it is suspected that a situation is getting or may get out of control, a supervisor should be notified without delay.

25. While on duty, lifeguards should provide their full name, position, and employer to any person requesting the information.

26. Lifeguards must never use foul language in the performance of their duty.

27. Lifeguards when not on duty are free to pursue their own course of action. However, they must keep in mind that they are representatives of their profession, their agency, and their community. Per-

sonal actions adverse to these responsibilities cannot be countenanced.

Lifeguards, together with personnel greeting individuals visiting agency offices and personnel going into the community to present the message the agency wishes to provide, are the three branches of any marine agency public relations program. These often interrelated and overlapping elements must be carefully monitored by the public relations staff. A PR program that covers two branches but not the third, is an incomplete program en route to disaster. All three branches of the agency staff need to be schooled in their relations with the public as part of an ongoing program instituted and subject to periodic review by the PR committee or staff.

Any public relations program, to be effective, must be tailored to the institution it serves. No two agencies, and therefore no two public relations programs, have precisely the same objectives, are directed to the same audience, or embrace identical tasks. The principles are the same, but the tools of communication will vary considerably. Good public relations is a good public service because it benefits the public. To this end, as Sidney J. Harris has stated so well, "Good public relations does not consist so much in telling the public as in listening to it. It provides a feedback that is otherwise lacking in the organizational structure."

That is the other side of the golden coin of public relations. Not only is the public informed of the mission of the marine agency, but the agency itself is informed by the public what its full mission might be. Public relations if practiced by the marine safety agency in this two-way fashion will serve as a continuing effort to create a harmonious adjustment between the agency and the public it serves. The adjustment is achieved by an exchange of information, of a give and take, that does not "just happen," but is planned and provided for by the agency public relations team.

The lifeguard on the beach, the agency director addressing a meeting of Boy Scout leaders, the secretary answering the telephone at the agency are all receiving unplanned and unprovided for input on how the public feels about the agency. This can be very helpful, but the public relations staff, in designing its program and in all its efforts, must provide for the planned input of public thoughts and thinking about the agency.

"Public relations," according to the prime minister of India, Mrs. Indira Ghandi, "is one of the lubricants of democracy. Governmental and industrial processes are becoming increasingly complex. It is through public relations that these processes can be made intelligible to the people and enable them to leave their impress on the shaping of policies." This is the mission of a marine safety agency public relations program—communication from government to citizen and from citizen to government. Public relations as practiced by the agency answers the question raised by Aristotle centuries ago: "The environment is complex and the political capacity of man is simple; can a bridge be built between them?"

3

Hazardous Water and Surf Conditions

The changing personality of the ocean is of vital concern to every marine safety guard. In 1847, the romantic American poet, Epes Sargent, wrote of the continually changing complexion of the sea:

A life on the ocean wave,
　A home on the rolling deep;
Where the scattered waters rave,
　And the winds their revels keep!
Like an eagle caged I pine
　On this dull, unchanging shore:
Oh, give me the flashing brine,
　The spray and the tempest's roar!

No lifeguards longs for stormy surf, but Sargent's poem does capture our fascination with the sea. The ocean surf provides an environment for aquatic sports and recreation completely different from the conditions found in bodies of still water such as bays, lakes, rivers, or manmade swimming pools. At sea, powerful forces generated by water movements are continuously at work. The surf, calm at one moment, can within hours become rough and dangerous. Even when the ocean floor is level at a given site, deep channels may lie to either side with fast rip currents running seaward through them. If the surf is calm, a single lifeguard can supervise hundreds of bathers successfully, but if there is "flashing brine" and "tempest's roar" and the surf is violent, several guards may experience difficulty safeguarding the same number of bathers.

With few exceptions, ocean waves are formed by winds and storms at sea. Changes in barometric pressure—high or low atmospheric pressure—cause pulsation by an entire storm system against the ocean surface, resulting in water movement. These wind-generated waves frequently travel across great expanses of water, thousands of miles of open sea, before breaking upon shore. Three factors affect wind generated waves—(1) wind velocity or speed; (2) distance traveled over open water (fetch); and (3) duration of the blow.

A wave is created when the frictional drag of a breeze on a calm sea causes ripples on its surface. Each of these ripples presents an angled surface against which the moving air exerts pressure. As the velocity of the wind increases, more water is moved, thus building the waves higher until their crests reach an angle of less than 120 degrees and the height of the wave is one-seventh of the length. When these conditions are met, the wave breaks at sea.

A set of waves, or wave trains, are incoming rows of waves characterized by four factors—(1) the period of time that it takes two consecutive wave crests to pass a given point; (2) the "wave length," which is the distance between the two crests; (3) the height of each crest above the trough or, conversely, the lowest point between the

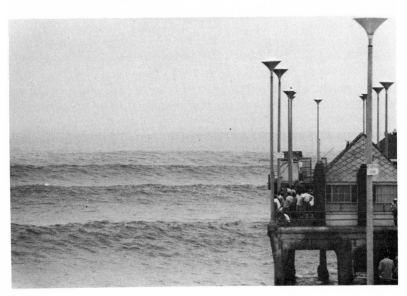

two crests; and (4) the velocity in knots at which the incoming set of waves advances or, colloquially, the speed of the wave train.

As ocean waves form and move out and away from the wind, their crests become more rounded and move in sets in which each wave is of a similar period and height. These wave trains are now called "ground swells" and can travel thousands of miles before they break on a distant shore. Swells, on almost any beach, come from a predictable direction that, unless altered by storm activity, changes with the seasons.

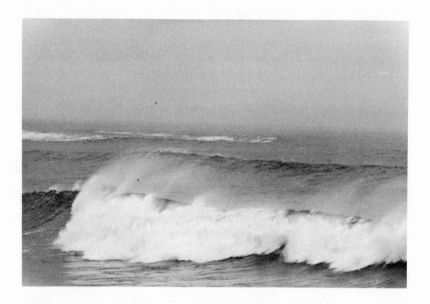

Since storms are erratic by nature, storm surf is erratic. Storm waves feature few lulls, and the waves come from many directions. For example, on the western shores of the United States, predominant swells originating at sea at latitudes as far south as 40 degrees in the southern Pacific continue to come from this southern ocean area from the middle of April until the first part of October. From early October to the middle of April, the swell direction changes, and the waves along the western coast originate in northern Pacific areas near the Aleutian Islands. California surfers call these waves, bursting with energy and power, "Aleutian juice." The changing source of these western coastal swells causes clearly visible visual changes in the beaches themselves. During the wintery northern drift, sand is lost from West Coast beaches, but in most cases is promptly replaced from its off-shore depository when the summer swells from the southern Pacific take over again.

Swells in the open sea are called surface waves if they are moving in water deeper than one-half their wave length. Surface waves move at speeds equal to three and a half times their wave period in seconds. For example, a wave with a period of ten seconds is travelling about thirty-five miles per hour, and this ten-second period is the average time between storm swells reaching the shores of the mainland United States.

The velocity of each wave is commensurably slowed as the water depth decreases. When this occurs, the surface waves become shallow water waves. As the wave trains approach the shoreline, the lengths decrease, wave heights increase, and velocities are reduced, but the periods remain unchanged. As the water depth decreases, the waves are refracted or bent to approximately the shape of the underlying ocean floor. As the water depth continues to decrease, the faster moving water at the crest spills over the slower moving water beneath; thus the waves break, and now parallel to the beach, they are termed surf. The remaining shoreward moving water—or *uprush*—runs onto the beach until its final energy is spent, and then it falls back into the sea.

The configuration of the ocean floor has a decisive influence on the manner in which a wave breaks. When a large swell is forced to expel its energy rapidly upon colliding with a steep underwater slope or reef, the crest of the wave tends to plunge or peak quickly, causing the water to mix with air and form foam or "white water." An ocean bottom that slopes gradually upward into shallows forms a wave that spills gently, with the small froth of white water being pushed ahead of the broken wave on its journey to the beach. These gentle waves create less sound than plunging waves that spray into the sky as air and water are trapped and compressed together. The experienced lifeguard knows how important the sound of waves in the darkness or in a fog can be to rescue work. Wave sounds can indicate to the lifesaver four vital conditions—(1) the type of wave that is breaking; (2) the power of the surf; (3) the location of the main break in the surf; and (4) the approximate width of the surf zone.

Anyone who has sat by the shore and surveyed the sea understands that no two waves are ever alike—similar, but never identical. For convenience, however, waves are classified into three primary forms—(1) *spilling waves,* which are formed by swells as they move over an ocean floor that ascends gradually beneath them, with the crest of the wave, when shallow water is reached, spilling onto the wave face until the wave itself is engulfed by foam; (2) *plunging waves,* which are formed when a swell suddenly strikes a shallow ocean bottom, reef, or other obstacle and breaks with flying spray, both expending most of its energy and transforming it into a spilling wave for its remaining distance to shore; and (3) *surging waves,* which occur where water is deep adjacent to shoreline cliffs, reefs, or steep beaches, with the wave keeping their trochoidal (i.e., water rotating in a circular motion) form until they crash against the shoreline barrier.

Waves are measured in different ways for different purposes. The space from trough to peak just before breaking differs from the front to the back of a given wave. The heights of the sides of incoming waves are of vital interest to lifeguards, who use this information to assess the turbulence of the surf and its potential effect on those in, on, or near the water. Unless waves can be measured against a nearby structure of known size, wave height is estimated by comparison to the body of a surfer as he stands erect on his surfboard or in relation to swimmers. Marine geologists and oceanographers generally agree that a wave breaks when the water depth is 1.3 times the visible height of the wave.

Very heavy surf can sometimes help lifeguards because the force of a succession of large breakers keeps swimmers and bathers close to shore, if not completely out of the water. However, during lulls—calm periods between successive sets—increasing numbers of beach patrons may venture further into the surf than they should, only to suffer when the big waves return.

This situation can be further aggravated by the fact that it is during such lulls, following immediately after sets, that rip currents and lateral drifts caused by the great volumes of water that have just been brought up to shore are the strongest. Such currents and drifts are actually waves above sea level seeking a return to the lower level of the sea from whence they came by rushing through any channel or depression in the sea floor—thereby generating a rip current. If beach patrons can be confined to safe areas during lulls by observant lifeguards, trouble will be minimized.

Backwash is noticeable on steeply inclined beaches during—or just before or just after—high tide. By definition, backwash occurs when the uprush of waves returning seaward gains momentum on the steep incline and returns with gathering force to the surf from whence it first came. When the surf is rough, a second uprush can meet the first uprush returning, creating extensive turbulence that is particularly dangerous to the elderly and very young people who may be in the shallow water near the shore. Often a backwash can create its own rip current, so that individuals knocked off their feet can be swept swiftly into deeper water.

Steep beaches are also subject to shore breaks. These are plunging waves that break in shallow water. Waves five to eight feet high or higher have been known to break in knee deep water during heavy surf conditions. When this occurs, a vigorous suction is caused both by the breaking wave and by the backwash from the previous wave. As a result of this seaward flow, a person standing in its grasp could be swept off his or her feet. If they are unfamiliar with the sea, they can be injured, and nonswimmers could actually drown under the weight of the oncoming waves. A person caught off balance in such a situation should push himself under and toward the oncoming wave, curl his body to withstand its force, and break out of this position on the other side of the wave. A tense, extended body, if hit by the full force of these waves, can suffer serious blows to the back and neck, and receive abrasions on the skin.

A lateral current, also known as a long shore current, usually runs parallel to the beach and perpendicular to the direction at which waves approach shore. This current may be so strong that a swimmer is unable to retain his position relative to the shore. Those who pay no attention can be swept sideways into a rip and then beyond the breakers.

Sandbars and troughs are found where a persistent lateral current has cut a channel into the ocean floor near the beach. The shapes of these channels vary, but they are sometimes as much as eight or ten feet deep and run hundreds of feet parallel to the shore before turning seaward. A single sandbar may exhibit several breaks, and a "rip current" may form at each break.

Rip currents occur when waves spilling over the sandbar and into the trough on the shoreward side pile up, then exit quickly through any break in the wall of sand that traps them. These troughs range from only a few feet to perhaps 150 feet wide. Water rushing along such a trough seeking a seaward outlet may move faster than a beach patron can swim, and even a wader may not be able to regain the safety of the shore against its pull. Sandbars can be attractive deceptions to a poor swimmer. Seeing bathers standing in shallow water far out from the shore, he may try to wade out, not realizing that deep water lies between himself and his goal, and thus may quickly find himself beyond his capacity to swim or cope with the current.

"Inshore holes" are depressions up to several yards in diameter dug into the sand by wave action at any depth, but often near shore. A small child can easily step from ankle deep water into depths over his head. These holes are as much a hazard to the lifeguard as they are to waders because he can sprain or fracture an ankle as he runs to make a rescue.

GENERAL TYPES OF RIP CURRENTS AND OTHER HAZARDS

Estimates of surf rescues caused by rip currents run as high as 80 percent. Even an expert swimmer can be almost helpless in the surf if he does not know what to expect. Rip currents actually attract swimmers because a flattening effect as the water rushes toward midocean causes the sea to look deceptively smooth at that location. If a swimmer is knowledgeable about rip currents and either avoids them, has learned how to swim out of them, or uses them to his advantage, little danger exists.

Rip currents vary in size, width, depth, shape, speed, and power. There are various causes of rip currents, but the most common are caused when torrents of water are brought to the beach in the form of waves. Since water seeks its own level, the excess water runs parallel to the beach away from the predominate swell direction until it finds a dip or hole in the ocean floor. Here the excess water turns seaward with little or no resistance because the deeper water in the hole has caused the waves running over it to flatten.

There are four general types of rip currents—(1) fixed, (2) permanent, (3) flash, and (4) traveling. Fixed rips are found only on sand beaches. They pull seaward in one location because the depth of the ocean floor directly underneath is greater than surrounding depths. These rips remain fixed in the same location so long as sand conditions remain stable in that section of the ocean floor. When surf conditions change, fixed rips may also change if the wave action subtracts or adds more sand to the hole. Therefore, a fixed rip may lie in a given spot one day, then change characteristics or simply disappear on the next day or on the next tide.

Permanent rips are stationary and are usually found on rocky coastlines. The excess water fed by the surf follows the contour of the rock formations seaward. The rock formations, which may be above the waterline or submerged, rarely change. Therefore, a seaward movement of the water in the same location may be expected everyday that waves are present. The speed and the power of these rips depend entirely on the size of the surf. Large surf feeds these rips a great volume of water, whereas small surf may hardly feed them at all. This same principle obviously applies to all rip currents, but is much more noticeable in the permanent type. Rock beach rip currents usually pull harder than sand beach rips because water moves more forcefully over solid, stationary obstacles, and the excess flow of water is more concentrated in the more pronounced rock channels.

Piers, rock jetties, drain pipes, projecting points of land, and some beach contours may also force lateral drifts to turn seaward, creating permanent rip currents. On occasion, a fixed rip will remain in one area for an entire season before disappearing and thus become known as a permanent rip due to its unusual endurance. Tidal outflows from bays and river and stream flows into the ocean are considered permanent rip currents.

The advantage for the lifeguard of permanent rip currents is that he can learn their characteristics and their habits, and rescues in them almost become routine. He can use them to reach a victim without delay, learn how to swim out of them while towing a victim, and utilize their power in different types of surf. Under these conditions, without hesitation, a lifeguard can know what rescue gear is needed and what backup assistance is required. It has been traditional for permanent rips or enduring fixed rips to be given names that relate to nearby landmarks or streets. Such identification can be invaluable when lifeguard teams answer emergency telephone calls because such names pinpoint where assistance is needed.

Flash rips are temporary rips and are generated by increased volumes of water brought to shore from sudden wave build-ups. Flash rips do not accompany depressions in the ocean floor very often. They usually occur during periods of irregular and stormy surf conditions or when the surf is heavy, with long lulls between sets of waves. Flash rips in the ocean, like flash floods on land, occur unexpectedly and without warning. When they strike an otherwise safe swimming area suddenly, part of the bathing crowd can be swept out toward the open sea. Many, since flash rips are always a temporary aquatic phenomenon, can return to shore without assistance, but those who are nonswimmers or who have panicked require rescuing. Since it is not always possible to decide from a station on the beach who is endangered by the flash rip, rescue operations must begin immediately, and usually several lifeguards are needed.

If flash rips occur repeatedly in the swimming area on a given day, that portion of the shore should be closed to water activities, or warnings should be issued periodically over the public address system to caution bathers to remain in shallow waters. There have been instances where a large group of bathers or a large mass of seaweed has caused a sudden lateral drift to turn seaward, forming a rip. When this phenomenon involves a group of bathers, part of the group may be drawn seaward.

Traveling rips do not accompany depressions in sand or reef formations. These rips are pushed up or down along a beach by the prevailing drag (lateral drift). Traveling rips usually occur in a strong, one-direction swell movement with long, well-defined periods. The lateral drift moves the rip away from the set of waves that feeds it. It usually continues moving and pulling well into the lull period following the particular wave set until the excess water has dissipated. The next set of waves starts the process all over again. These rips can be pushed 200 to 300 yards and further along the beach, depending on the size of the surf and/or the number of waves in a set. They are similar in all respects to flash rips except that their movement is predictable once their sequence has begun, and the established pattern repeats itself.

CHARACTERISTICS OF RIP CURRENTS

Although rip currents can vary greatly in appearance, as a general rule they look in some way distinctly different from the surrounding surf. A rip may seem especially rough or choppy, may have the dark color of water deeper than that on either side of it, and may or may not have foam. Rips sometimes pick up debris, kelp particles, or sand from the ocean floor, giving the water a dirty or muddy quality; other times the seaward current shows clear evidence that the water at the surface is running in the opposite direction from the incoming waves and is either flowing perpendicular to them or at any other angle from the shore. A rip moving through a calm, level surf is easily detected. They are harder to spot when the sea is rough and conditions are windy. Under any conditions, a rip can be seen easily from a high elevation overlooking the surfline.

Fixed and permanent rips pull the hardest, as a general rule, when tides are lowest. This is because the rip channels are deeper and more definite compared to the surrounding areas, which are at their shallowest. Consequently, the excess water is considerably more concentrated into the channels while returning seaward. It is also true that all rip currents pull the hardest during the lull immediately following a set of waves. This is because with the absence of any incoming waves, the excess water volume has complete freedom on its return to the sea. Certain rips characteristically stop pulling at high tide, only to begin again at low tide; and the reverse situation is also possible. Because of all these changing rip conditions, the lifeguard must constantly read the surfline in order to safeguard his assigned area of responsibility.

The most difficult rip currents to swim out of are rock rips. Areas bordering the main rip hole are often shallow and filled with jagged rocks covered by shell fish and barnacles. These shallow waters can lacerate a swimmer seeking the shore and deliver severe abrasions. For a lifeguard with a rescue victim these difficulties are accentuated. A "landline" can be very useful for rescuing persons from the neck of a rock beach rip and bringing them to the beach. With the landline, the victim can be towed through deep water where chances for injury are minimal and guided away from sharp reefs at the sides of the neck or from other rocks and sea growths along the rescue route. The only alternatives are to swim to another point of access to the beach or wait outside the surfline for a rescue vessel or helicopter.

Statistically, spring and early summer are the most hazardous times on the western beaches of the American shoreline because of the unstable condition of the offshore ocean floor—a condition caused by the irregular bottom condition and created primarily by winter storms. These conditions, further aggravated by cold waters and swimmers physically out of condition, can make the job of the lifeguard appreciably more difficult during the first warm weather periods of spring.

As spring and summer progress, milder swells usually tend to level the sandy ocean floor, making the bottom considerably less threatening to beach patrons, but mild seasons often have rough water periods from tropical storm centers that are dangerous for beach goers. At any time, swimming against the seaward current of a rip is difficult, and at times impossible, even for the strongest swimmers, as well as for swimmers using fins, surfers paddling their surfboards, or patrons using flotation devices. Some bathers enter rips because they are unaware of their existence or ignorant of their dangers. Others frequently enter the water at a safe location but are swept along with the lateral drag into a rip.

All rip currents are broken down into three components—feeder, neck, and head. The feeder is the main source of supply for the rip. A rip current may have one or two feeders. For example, waves breaking on both sides of a deeper water channel would create two feeders. Single-feeder rip currents are, however, much more common. A feeder is actually the lateral drift—the side current—of water brought to shore by the waves, which in turn seek a means of returning to the level of the sea.

The neck portion of a rip current is the river of water running seaward. The neck can vary in width from a few yards to several hundred yards. The majority of rescues and the majority of drownings occur in the neck. The simplest way for a swimmer to escape from the seaward pull of the neck is to swim parallel to the beach.

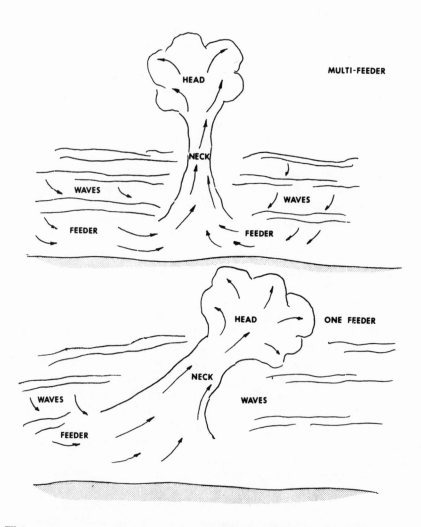

This maneuver is easy if the rip current is a stationary one, but if it is a traveling rip moving in the same direction as the swimmer, then an attempt to escape its force can be futile. Swimmers may also enter the feeder zone and be sucked into the neck, as these rip currents may flow faster than the swimmer can swim.

Considering the seriousness and number of rip hazards, it is clear that any swimmer should stop, look, and study a rip before making his or her move. If the main feeder zone must be crossed in order to reach shore, one should either swim a good distance away from the neck or be prepared to swim hard across the feeder by using the swell and wave action for forward movement while avoiding the

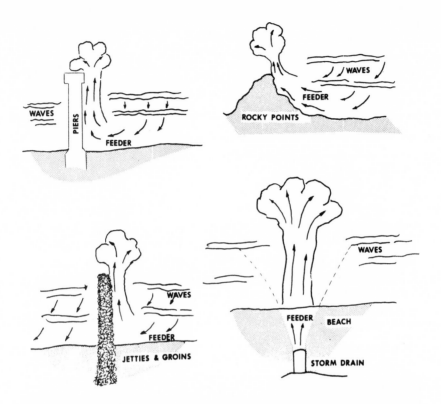

neck. A rip current can also be escaped when the swimmer relaxes and allows it to carry him to its outermost limit—its head—which is usually not far beyond the breakers where surfers congregate to await their choice of waves to ride. After judging the width of the rip current, the swimmer can swim parallel to the beach in relatively calm water, reenter the surf, and then swim safely to shore.

4

Facilities and Equipment

BASIC FACILITIES

The basic lifeguard facility must start with the headquarters, the administrative facility, the heart of the lifesaving enterprise. The vast majority of marine safety agency activities and lifesaving functions are centered in a centralized administrative facility. These large, often multistory structures are usually located at the beach or bay front, with direct access to the marine environment they service, and incorporate administrative staff offices, communication and reception areas, first aid and recovery rooms, locker and shower facilities, training and apparatus room, maintenance shop, vehicle and equipment storage, meeting rooms, and often kitchen facilities.

If the marine safety agency's responsibilities are spread over a large and varied geographical area, there may be a number of secondary auxiliary quarters and facilities. Such decentralization is almost mandatory when widespread areas cannot feasibly be serviced by a single primary headquarters building. In this case, secondary facilities such as lifeguard beach headquarters, harbor facilities for rescue boats, substations, central vantage towers, and field patrol towers may be incorporated into the system.

The lifeguard beach headquarters is invariably located on a

strand of beach, in a cove, or on a bay and can easily serve as a main headquarters facility for much smaller marine safety services. These structures are outfitted with facilities for communications, observations, reception, information, lockers, showers, and limited vehicle and equipment storage. From the headquarters all personnel are deployed, emergency backup is available, and the treatment of medical needs monitored.

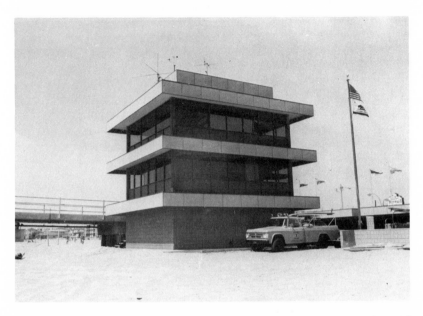

The primary safety service of a harbor facility for rescue boats is to control boat traffic in bay and harbor areas. Such a harbor facility usually houses sophisticated marine communications; observation, reception, and information areas; a limited medical aid facility; locker and shower area; workshop; boat hoists; and docking and fueling facilities for rescue boats, harbor patrol boats, and fire boats.

Substations are permanent two-story buildings located on outlying beaches, bays, or coves where high density beach patron visitation is experienced. Substations serve multiple functions. The top floor usually houses lifesaving observation, communication, reception, and information capacities. A public address system is also often located here. The ground floor may have vehicle storage and a medical aid area. A substation is an immediate source of primary backup to field patrol towers.

Marine safety agency operations that have a pier usually incorporate use of a central vantage tower strategically located on the pier.

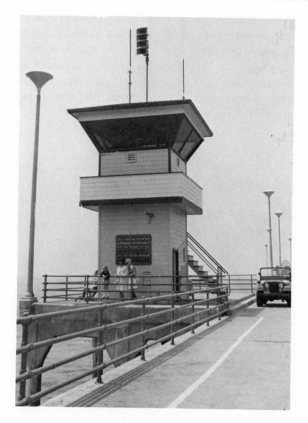

These elevated towers serve as a backup for every field patrol tower within observational limits. Central vantage towers provide considerable operational efficiency since they can have telephone or radio contact with other towers, vehicles, and boats, while the lofty observation platform allows an overview of the "perimeter defense system." Further, a high-powered public address system can be used to implement preventive lifeguarding.

Field patrol towers are the main ingredient in the "perimeter defense system" employed in the United States as the main method of lifesaving. These elevated towers may come in varied shapes and designs but they all function similarly. Depending on the environmental and geographical demands of the area, towers are strategically placed on beaches, bays, and coves. Field patrol towers can and do provide primary response to all waterfront emergencies. They must always be provided with tower-to-tower and tower-to-headquarters telephonic communication.

Some ocean lifeguard towers are open, but most modern ones are enclosed to protect the lifeguard from the elements and to provide some comfort during long hours on duty. Construction and design vary from area to area, but a minimum of six feet should be required, and towers should have glass fronts and sides that can be shuttered. Ladders or ramps for easy entry and expedient exit are essential. If properly constructed, towers can be securely shuttered and locked during off-duty or off-season periods. All towers must have adequate space for rescue and first aid gear as well as communication equipment.

Lifeguard emergency vehicles—the lifeguard mobile unit—have a fundamental and basic purpose—to provide needed specialized equipment in a specific area when the need arises, thereby eliminating the cost of duplicating equipment and manpower in each tower. Mobile units also provide transport to critical rescue areas. These units are manned by experienced guards or supervisory personnel who have the accumulated experience needed when a crisis requires sound judgment and an authoritative voice in a command position.

When utilizing lifeguard emergency vehicles, these general operating instructions should be followed:

1. Hard Surface Driving
   a. Be sure to use two-wheel drive at all times. Using four-wheel drive on hard surfaces results in undue strain on drive train components.
   b. When it is necessary to jump curbs upon entering the beach, do so slowly and use four-wheel drive.
   c. Do not make sharp or quick corner turns under any circumstances.
2. Sand Driving
   a. If locking mechanisms are present, be sure that front wheel hubs are in the lock position.
   b Use four-wheel drive at all times except on hard, packed sand.
   c. Use a gear combination that will keep the vacuum gauge out of the red zone. The vacuum gauge tells the operator how hard the engine is working.
   d. Do not ride the clutch or slip it more than is absolutely necessary.
   e. Check tire pressure regularly to guarantee that it remains at the correct pressure for sand driving. If the unit bogs down in soft sand, the pressure can be somewhat lowered.
   f. Be constantly alert for debris or holes on the beach that could damage the mobile unit.
   g. If the unit becomes stuck in the sand, alert headquarters at once so that beach coverage can be maintained otherwise and assistance can be dispatched.
   h. Be constantly alert for children. Children move rapidly and unpredictably, and they have no reason to expect a mobile unit on the beach.
   i. Avoid driving vehicles into any depressions of salt water during periods of low tide.
   j. Avoid driving units in the surf uprush when patroling below the berm—the point where the wet sand meets the dry sand.
   k. Do not accelerate through the gears or speed shift.
   l. Do not decelerate by using the gears.

m. Always engage the emergency brake when leaving the vehicle.
n. On a steep incline or soft sand, do not slip the clutch, use a lower gear or back up and attain more speed. The clutch should be fully engaged when driving.
o. Before placing a parked or temporarily stopped vehicle in motion, check underneath both the rear and front tires and under the carriage as well to make absolutely sure there are no obstructions in the pathway, whether materials, animals, or humans.
p. When maneuvering any marine safety vehicle in a tight area and/ or when visibility is impaired, it is the responsibility of the driver to have one of the other men in the unit direct him from outside the vehicle whenever possible. Extreme caution should be used at all times, especially when operating a vehicle with a trailer, large bed, or similar object extending beyond the normal length or width of the vehicle.

Marine safety agencies invariably develop patrol procedures germane to local conditions. In general, normal patrol procedures are:

1. Drive carefully and slowly unless responding to a call.
2. Do not drive closer than is absolutely necessary to any person or personal belongings.
3. Avoid conversation with the public unless necessary.
4. When stopping to answer questions or when giving guards a swim break, point the vehicle toward the ocean for constant water surveillance.
5. Do not stop at liquor stores for food snacks.
6. When the vehicle is parked at the edge of the berm, it is mandatory that the operator visually take whatever precautionary measures are necessary, such as getting physically out of the unit to determine that the path is clear of all persons or small children prior to driving the vehicle up the profile to the level berm.

This point is even more important in emergency circumstances because the operator is usually focused on the emergency zone and tends to be in a hurry thus not as cautious as he normally would be.

7. During the period of steep berm profile, avoid driving below the berm. This practice will insure that you will always be able to respond directly to a call rather than backtracking.
8. Do not permit unauthorized personnel to ride in the unit.
9. Conduct yourself in a businesslike manner at all times.
10. When relieving tower guards:
    a. Remain in radio contact unless the dispatcher is notified of your inability to monitor the air;
    b. Keep one man in the tower at all times; and
    c. Keep area in front of the tower clear to allow rapid exit.

Emergency call procedures differ from normal patrol procedures. In general emergency call procedures are:

1. Turn radio volume up.
2. Drive as fast as conditions will permit. Be especially careful at intersections. Stop at stop signs and red lights momentarily to be sure the area is clear.
3. Notify headquarters upon arrival at emergency location and advise headquarters as soon as possible as to what has happened and whether additional men or supplies are needed.
4. When 10-97 on an inclined berm, without fail set the emergency brake. Vehicle can be parked parallel to the ocean.
5. During emergency calls, red lights and sirens are used only when necessary. Under no circumstances, however, should sole reliance for clearing traffic be placed on red lights or sirens.
6. When involved in a Code III call on the beach, utilize good judgment.

Maintenance of mobile unit equipment is of vital importance. Any preshift checkout should include:

1. Check gas, oil, battery, and water;
2. Check radio, red lights, and sirens;
3. Check resuscitator and rescue equipment;
4. Check first aid supplies; and
5. Check forms and miscellaneous gear.

Postshift maintenance checking should include:

1. Refill vehicle with gasoline;
2. Check oil, battery, and water; and
3. Wash the vehicle, clean the interior using whisk broom on floorboards. Dry all chrome fixtures well.

Mobile safety vehicles must be serviced at regular, predetermined intervals. It is the responsibility of the vehicle driver to schedule servicing when it is due. Any damage or malfunction to vehicles must be reported to headquarters without delay.

Procedures if and when an accident with the vehicle takes places are:

1. Contact the local police;
2. Contact headquarters;
3. Leave vehicle in the exact area of the accident;
4. Make no statements except as necessary to police; and
5. Make out department vehicle accident reports.

Suggested minimum standard equipment for both call cars and beach units follow. For call cars:

1. A resuscitator plus four spare oxygen bottles;
2. Two pairs of fins;
3. Three masks with snorkels;
4. Four rescue cans;
5. One rescue board;

6. One backboard with straps (Velcro fasteners);
7. Boat tows;
8. Carrier;
9. Strobe light for night operations;
10. Flashlight;
11. Underwater flashlight;
12. Three blankets, rolled;
13. A large first aid kit;
14. A small first aid kit;
15. A bolt cutter;
16. Report-writing materials;
17. Binoculars;
18. Body bag;
19. Two splints—inflatable, cardboard, or other;
20. A pair of hand gloves;
21. Battery jumper cables; and
22. A fifteen-foot vehicle towline.

For beach units:

1. A resuscitator plus two spare oxygen bottles;
2. A pair of fins;
3. A mask with snorkel;
4. Two rescue cans;
5. A boat tow;
6. A small first aid kit;
7. Battery jumper cables;
8. Underwater flashlight;
9. Report-writing materials;
10. A fifteen-foot vehicle towline;
11. Two blankets;
12. A rescue tube;
13. A rescue board;
14. Two splints—inflatable, cardboard, or other; and
15. One stretcher.

Emergency vehicles should be easily identifiable. This can best be achieved by painting them with an outstanding color easily seen on the beach or in traffic. Three popular colors for marine safety agency vehicles are red, yellow, and international orange. Easy identification facilitates easy spotting by the tower lifeguards, rescue vessels, helicopters, and other backup units. A bright color also helps make the public aware of the presence of a vehicle on the beach and is an additional safety factor during an emergency call.

Electronic sirens have proven to be the most audible and draw less on batteries. Red emergency lights should be elevated above the windshield and face forward and should be either flashing or rotating. The rear emergency lights should be a blinking amber color, facing to the rear and above the rear windows.

Suggested equipment for rescue vessels, both the twin-screw rescue boat and the jet boat, follows, including maintenance procedures. First, the twin-screw rescue boat:

1. PA system;
2. Rescue tubes;
3. Towlines;
4. First aid kits;
5. Splints;
6. Fire extinguishers;
7. Salvage pump;
8. Fire pump;
9. Fire hoses;

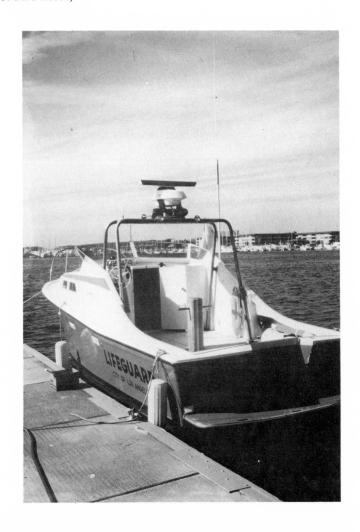

10. Radios;
11. Fire axe;
12. Resuscitators;
13. Blankets;
14. Diving (scuba) gear;
15. Battery jumper cables;
16. Bolt cutters;
17. Stretchers;
18. Market buoys;
19. Hull patch kits;
20. DCP radar;
21. Depth finder; and
22. Depth direction finder.

Proper and efficient maintenance cannot be overemphasized. The rescue vessel should be cleaned and polished in the morning before going on patrol or being placed in service. In the evening, the rescue boat should be hosed down to remove all salt water. The following maintenance schedule should keep the rescue boat in good working order:

1. Daily starting
   a. Open engine hatches and/or start blowers (gas engines);
   b. Check oil;
   c. Check fresh water in cooling system;
   d. Check fuel;
   e. Check transmission fluid;
   f. Start engines;
   g. Check gauges;
   h. Turn on radios and check;
   i. Check PA system; and
   j. Check all electrical systems.
2. Equipment requiring periodic checks
   a. Salvage pump and hoses;
   b. Resuscitator;
   c. Depth finder;
   d. Fire extinguishers;
   e. Rescue tubes;
   f. Diving equipment;
   g. First aid supplies;
   h. Towline;
   i. Boat hook and fire axe
   j. Foul weather gear;
   k. Compass;
   l. Life jackets;
   m. Anchor, chains, line;
   n. Blankets and stretchers;
   o. Flashlights;
   p. Navigation equipment; and
   q. Communication equipment.

3. Cleaning
   a. Brush off growth from bottom;
   b. Wash off inside, outside hull sides;
   c. Wash bilge and rinse with salt water;
   d. Chamois off boat;
   e. Polish all bright work; and
   f. Clean all radio antennas.
4. Monthly maintenance
   a. Grease steering mechanisms and other necessary moving parts;
   b. Grease throttle and shifting linkage;
   c. Drain fuel water trap and clean filter;
   d. Clean flame arresters;
   e. Check batteries with hydrometer and connections;
   f. Check engine zinc plates and engine zincs;
   g. Check hull packing glands;
   h. Clean salt water strainer as needed;
   i. Check fittings and bolts; and
   j. Change oil and filters.

The jet boat, the newest innovation in surf rescue boats, has many advantages over more convention craft. It (1) is capable of entrance and exit through very rough surf conditions; (2) can operate inside the surf zone; (3) is highly maneuverable, with fast acceleration and deceleration; (4) can turn 180 degrees within its own wake; and (5) has a smooth bottom with no propellers, which allows operation in very shallow water and eliminates the problem of electrolysis.

While these superb capabilities make the jet boat a more functional rescue craft both in remote areas that are virtually inaccessible to land units and in semi remote areas where water population is minimal, there are certain disadvantages in heavy rescue activity areas. For example, the jet boat (1) is a single engine craft and, if it loses power inside the surfline, has no auxiliary engine; (2) cannot maintain as stable a position when working critical rescue operations; (3) has less room on board for rescue victims; and (4) has a flat bottom design that makes it extremely difficult to maintain a steady course in rough seas.

The jet ski is the very latest innovation in surf rescue equipment. While its capabilities on prime activity days are severely limited due to its size and virtually nonexistent capacity for securing rescue gear and equipment, the jet ski can provide invaluable service during early morning and late evening hours and throughout the off-season months, especially when personnel are at a minimum, and the rescue vessels are not on patrol.

The major advantages of the jet ski are (1) it can be transported to the scene quickly in a moderate size emergency backup vehicle by two persons: (2) it takes only one lifeguard to operate; (3) maintenance and operation costs are minimal; (4) if the operator falls off or is thrown off, it automatically idles in a 360 degree rotation; and (5) it can be operated in and around the surf zone at minimal hazard to either operator or swimmers.

BASIC RESCUE EQUIPMENT

The most widely used rescue gear in the ocean environment are the lifeguard rescue tube and rescue buoy. They can, however, be used successfully in any water environment. The rescue tube is a flexible buoy of polyurethane foam, thirty-eight by six by three inches, tapering to a one-inch wide, rubber-coated canvas strap at one end of the tube. The other end is equipped with an external rubber-coated canvas strap, ten inches by one inch, with two brass rings attached. There are a wide variety of rescue tubes available on the market. Older types that were inflated by air are being phased out because of the danger of puncture. A disadvantage of the rubber rescue tube is its buoyancy, which severely limits its effectiveness when two or more victims are being rescued.

The rescue buoy was originally torpedo shaped and was constructed from sheet steel, and later from spun aluminum. The great surfer from Hawaii, George Freeth, who had been brought to California to be its first lifeguard by the late land magnate, Henry E. Huntington, traditionally is credited with the invention of the rescue buoy. The latest and most functional rescue buoys are constructed of synthetic polyurethane, which provides smoother angles all around, and in some cases they have molded handles for

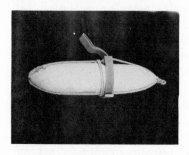

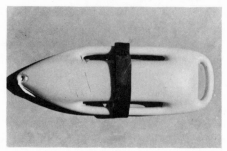

victims to grasp and hang onto. Earlier models had a line attached around the buoy for the support of victims.

In most instances, rescue buoys and rescue tubes are attached to six-foot lines with either a canvas or nylon strap on the end opposite to slip over the lifeguard's shoulder or a belt to slip around the guard's waist. This design permits the rescuer to swim freely through the water, towing the buoy and rescued victim behind. When on duty, the lifeguard keeps the rescue tube or buoy close at hand with the strap and rope wrapped for quick release. When the rubber tube is stored for long periods of time, the line should hang free, as tight strapping during storage tends to deform the tube.

Care of rescue buoys is important. For those made from spun aluminum the chance of puncture is slim, but it does exist. Rescue buoys must be checked thoroughly after any rescue where it may have been bumped or used as a fending device. Its paint should be refreshed at least once yearly for easy visibility, to protect its surface, and to keep it attractive. No buoy should be made of material that will rust. Plastic fiberglass buoys occasionally crack after rough treatment and must be inspected regularly. Rubber rescue buoys need very little maintenance other than storage in a shaded area to prevent eventual sun rot. Each buoy should be numbered to assist with inventory procedures, and numbers can be assigned both to specific stations and to individual guards. This permits each guard to know that the belt or harness attached to the buoy is the best type for him and fits properly. Both plastic and rubber buoys are manufactured with the color pigmented into the material.

All buoy lines need regular inspection and should be replaced at the first sign of rot, fraying, or a possible break. Any line of substantial strength is satisfactory and should have a diameter no larger than three-eighths and not less than one-fourth of an inch. Recommended line materials are polypropylene, three strand or braided strand; nylon three strand; or manila.

The landline is not in general use today, but it is still used in some areas. If it is used, the lifeguard attaches a belt around his waist that is secured to a line that feeds out from a large reel on the beach. The reel can be manned by one three-man team, or it can be secured on an emergency vehicle or to some object on land. On the beach, smaller reels can be used with smaller crews.

When the lifeguard reaches the victim, he signals by hand, and the men on shore wind the reel, pulling the rescuer and victim to shore. It is important that the reel be carefully wound to avoid dangling loops that could cause a severe backlash. The landline has proven to be highly impractical in crowded areas or if used near piers, wharfs, groins, jetties, and other aquatic structures. This is because strong drifts can cause the line to tangle when encountering obstructions, plus the every present possibility of endangering other bathers and swimmers on return.

The rescue board is one of many tools from which the lifeguard can choose to suit a particular emergency. The rescue board fills the gap between the rescue buoy and the surf rescue boat. The rescue board is a paddleboard—the paddleboard originally conceived and designed by Thomas C. Blake, the All-American swimmer turned surfer who became a close friend to Duke Paoa Kahanamoku and invented the skeg used on all surfboards today.

The use of the rescue board, or rescue paddleboard, is limited by its accessibility as well by surf conditions, but it can enable a lifeguard to execute an efficient rescue considering the alternatives at any given moment. Its advantages are:

1. Speed and conserved energy. A rescue board allows the lifeguard to travel long distances much more quickly and with less effort than swimming. Once the lifeguard has reached and recovered the victim, he can return to shore with the victim aboard the deck of the rescue board much more swiftly than possible while swimming. A conscious victim may also be able to contribute to the paddling and thereby enhance the speed of the return.

2. Portability. A rescue board is easily handled by one lifeguard alone and can be readily moved almost anyplace a single guard can go. From piers, bridges, jetties, or low cliffs, the rescue board can be either dropped or lowered. A rescue boat or mobile unit on land can carry a board. It can be stored in or next to an observation tower ready for immediate use. It will float in water too shallow for boats or swimmers and can ride a lifeguard over kelp too thick to swim through if its fin is properly designed.

3. Flotation. A rescue board is buoyant enough to support a number of nonpanicked victims at the same time. If offers the rescuing lifeguard a fairly stable area on which to work with an asphyxiated or seriously injured victim. It can also carry a heavy person, a person weighted by a scuba or surfing wetsuit, or a heavily clothed victim with more ease than a conventional rescue buoy.

4. Visibility. Because of the height attained while knee paddling a rescue board, the lifeguard can maintain visual contact with a victim while simultaneously observing any hazards, currents, or approaching waves much better than if he were swimming.

Disadvantages are:

1. Proportional loss of control. A rescue board is difficult, if not impossible, to move through heavy surf. A swimming lifeguard can penetrate such surf, while a rescue board cannot. Trying to return to shore with a frightened or incapacitated victim is arduous in sizeable surf. Loss of the rescue board itself in the surf is the gravest danger. If the board is lost, the lifeguard is left without equipment and could

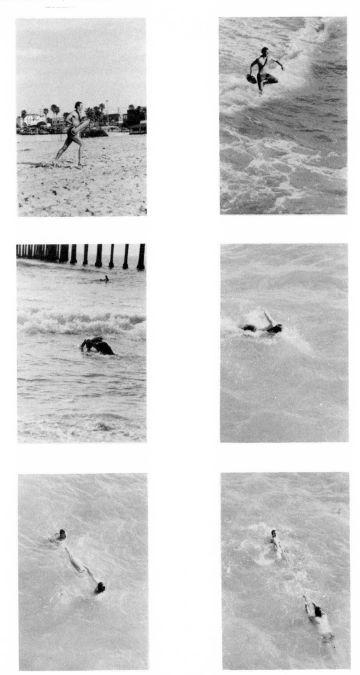

lose visual contact with the victim. Congested swimming areas, for this reason, must be avoided when making board rescues.

2. Material and/or design weaknesses. A rescue board is easily damaged and is in constant need of repair. Unrepaired deck surfaces can cause injury to both lifeguards and victims. Rescue boards are awkward to use, and unless sufficient time has been devoted to learning the necessary skills, only highly trained personnel can utilize the board rescue.

Desired design specifications for the Blake rescue board follow:

1. Design and buoyancy factors. A rescue board is a buoyant board that is fast and maneuverable through still water and low surf, comfortable to handle on land, and large enough to accommodate two people at sea, even if one of the two individuals is weighted with clothing or gear.
2. Bottom design. Flat bottoms are the fastest and the most stable. Convex or concave rescue board bottoms are undesirable.
3. Rails or edges. "Round" or "downed" (half-moon-shaped) rails are apparently more stable than other designs.
4. Rocker/spoon or kick. "Rocker" means that the center portion of the back of the board is lower than the nose or tail block, and "kick" refers to the curve in the nose. Boards having little or no rocker are susceptible to purling. Controlling a "straight" or "flat" board is very difficult because of this characteristic.
5. Tail block or stern. A pointed flat tail block is probably the fastest design, but the most unstable at paddling speeds. A wide, flat tail block seems the most stable for paddling, so rescue boards are a compromise between the two design concepts.
6. Buoyancy. Since a rescue board must be capable of rapid propulsion while loaded with victim and rescuer, any board falling short of this achievement would be inadequate.
7. Length. Most boards now in use are about eleven to twelve feet in length, with weight averaging twenty-five to forty pounds.
8. Width. Current preferred widths are twenty-three to twenty-four inches. Less width means less stability; more width reduces maneuverability in the water and increases awkwardness when carried on land.
9. Thickness. Currently three to four inches at the thickest part of the rescue board is considered best; anything thinner would sacrifice buoyancy.
10. Colors. A rescue board should be pigmented or brightly colored so that rescue operations can be easily followed. As in other rescue equipment, those colors most easily identifiable from beach, air, or water are international (or Coast Guard) orange, tahiti or bright yellow, and signal or bright red. Functional coloring of the fin (skeg) should also be considered. A rescue board that is accidentally lost in the water is often flipped bottom up and can be recovered by the guard in the water if the fin color is a prominent one. During turbulent surf conditions, where the board is only glimpsed between waves, black, dark blue, dark brown, and dark red are acceptable fin colors.

11. Handles. Rope handles can be installed on rescue boards to assure better control and increase versatility. For example, with handles, the rescue board can be used easily as a stretcher. An eyelet on the bottom of the nose also aids towing.

12. Construction materials. Today most rescue boards are manufactured from a shaped reinforced core of polyurethane foam and then covered with a skin of fiberglass and pigmented resins, a concept borrowed from the modern surfboard first created by the late Robert Simmons while studying at the California Institute of Technology.

13. Types of fins or skegs. Fin design noticeably affects board performance in the ocean environment. A fin with a large surface area, about eight inches deep and ten inches at the base and having an obtuse dorsal shape, is more stable than a small, sickle-shaped fin. Although a small fin offers greater maneuverability and ease of turning, the board is more difficult to control. A heavy kelp will catch a deep fin and hold it. The slanted leading edge of a "kelp skeg" reduces this problem. Shallow reefs or shelflike rocky shorelines collide with deep board fins, making control difficult and forward progress slow. Strong side currents complicate the situation. Under these circumstances, the shorter the fin, the better, yet reduction of fin surface area and depth causes proportional loss of stability and board control. A possible compromise is the use of two small "twin fins"—one to each rail and parallel, with slanted leading edges for kelp penetration. The removable skeg in a fin box, the refinement and invention of Hobart "Hobie" Alter, tandem surfer and boat enthusiast, is desirable both for multipurpose use of the board and ease of replacement or repair. These "slow" or "box" type fins are available in a kaleidoscope of colors, sizes, and designs.

The maintenance, repair, wear, and waxing of rescue boards deserves specific attention. The polyurethane board is stronger than former board materials but it is not indestructible. It is very vulnerable to sharp blows, constant heavy pressure, sunlight, and, if penetrated, to waterlogging and rot. The key to maintaining a rescue board in good shape and ready for action is *preventive* care. Protection from abuse can prolong its life and reduce repair costs. An adequate place for board storage is a must. Periodic washing, preferably at the end of each day, removes salts that attract moisture and can combine with sunlight to hasten deterioration. Boards stored on rescue vehicles should be cleaned regularly to remove road grease that could hamper rescue efforts by making the board slippery. During normal usage, a polyurethane rescue board is subject to breaks in the fiberglass covering—or "dings" as the surfing community calls them. The result of neglected dings is discoloration, waterlogging, and eventual separation of the fiberglass covering from the foam core.

In general, a rescue board will receive the most wear along its rails near the tail block, caused by the manner it is dragged through the sand by a lifeguard running to make a rescue. Although this abrasion is difficult to prevent, lifeguards should refrain from dragging boards. When the wind is still enough so that a carried board can be controlled, a lifeguard should run with the center of the board tucked under his arm, as surfers do, to prevent it from touching the ground.

Paraffin wax is applied to the surface of a polyurethane rescue board to provide traction and to create a nonslip deck surface. Never have waxes been developed specifically for this purpose. Paraffin melts easy, rubs off, and must be replaced often. Mixtures are available that do not melt in hot weather or warm water and maintain their nonslip characteristics in cold environments as well. Wax should be maintained on the board at all times, and the best way to apply it is by hand in a circular fashion.

A rescue board should be stored for easy access. It must be kept where it can be reached without delay at all times. When not in use, the board should be stored close to the water in a safe situation where it will not be damaged. A path leading from the rescue board to entry into the water should be kept clear at all times. At night, or when the lifeguard station is closed, the board should be kept in a place especially provided for storage to facilitate quick location in the event of an emergency. On emergency vehicles or rescue crafts, a padded rack can be devised to keep obstruction to a minimum. This will permit securing the board so it will not slip off while providing for quick release should the board be needed suddenly. One example of an adequate fastener is the heavy duty rubber cord. Always store boards wax side down to protect the wax from sunlight.

Each lifeguard has his own personal equipment—swim fins, sunglasses, binoculars, and whistles. The adjustable strap and "shoe" fins are inadequate in the surf because they have a tendency to come off and are therefore not recommended for lifeguarding. A good pair of fins provides speed, power, and added protection for the feet. On routine sand beach rescues, where the victims are usually a short distance from the shore, fins are a nuisance and time consuming since the lifeguard has to stop to put them on, but they can be a great advantage during a mass rescue when the guard must swim one hundred yards or more. Another advantage of fins is the arm freedom they provide since they add power to the guard's kick. Fins also permit better control of a victim when the rescuer and rescued are being hit by waves and white water.

When utilizing fins on rescues it is good to remember that (1) they are not designed for walking or running and if you try you may trip and injure yourself; and (2) for sloping sand beach rescues, fins should not be put on until the guard must start swimming. This is because they can slow a guard down and tend to cramp the legs and feet. Fins should be put on at a slow and steady pace. The few extra seconds taken to put them on correctly will be fully compensated for by the added power they will provide. Fins worm upside down tend to come off.

For rock beach rescue work in shallow water, fins are recommended as foot protection. This is the only time one should run with fins on. To avoid tripping, a high stride must be used. A guard should not wear the fins of another guard on rescues, as the fins may not fit. If too small, they will cause foot cramps, and if too large they may come off in the surf, leaving the rescuer helpless. Giant fins can cause leg cramps if one is not accustomed to them.

Sunglasses is a very important piece of equipment for a lifeguard. They not only protect the eyes, but allow a guard to see objects in the water that he would not be able to see without them. The constant glare of the water may ruin the eyes in one season without adequate protection. An optometrist should be consulted when obtaining sunglasses. Plastic ones are not recommended as they scratch easily.

Binoculars are valuable in areas where the lifeguard must cover a large body of water. By using binoculars, the lifeguard will be able to see clearly the actions and facial expressions of the swimmers and be able to determine who is in trouble and what type of rescue or preventive action is needed. Binoculars should be standard pieces of equipment in rescue boats and land rescue vehicles. Binocular lenses designed for night use with powers of 7 x 50 or 7 x 35 wide angle are highly recommended.

Whistles are predominantly used by lifeguards at swimming pools or in confined areas where they can be easily heard. They are used to alert patrons when they are violating rules and regulations. They can also be used by unit guards for communicating with tower guards in emergency situations.

5

Basic Rescue Techniques and Special Procedures

RECOGNIZING DISTRESSED SWIMMERS AND BATHERS

As a lifeguard gains experience, he often instinctively makes a correct rescue without fully comprehending what precise factors caused him to judge one situation dangerous and another safe. Seldom is the warning of trouble anything more than visual recognition of distress by an alert and experienced guard. The chatter of children playing, the commotion of people around the station, and the noise of the surf, muffles calls for help. There are many signs, however, that indicate to the guard that he is needed and that direct his attention to one afflicted person in a crowd of active swimmers or to someone alone in a remote location.

1. Facing the beach is a major signal given by possible victims as they direct themselves toward the safe place they wish to reach. If their progress is poor, they are floundering, their swimming stroke is weak, they are struggling to float, or their behavior is unnatural, they are probably in trouble. Swimmers doing a 360 degree turn in the water are often looking for the nearest exit or help. Close proximity of two swimmers may be nothing more than companionship, yet one or both may be seeking assistance desperately. A scuba diver with his faceplate and mouthpiece out of position may be gasping for air. When paddling a float, a swimmer may accidentally either fall or jump off or decide that he can swim faster than he can paddle, not realizing that a rip

current is pushing against him. The swimmer, making no forward progress as he heads beachward or even being pushed out to sea by the backwash, may become exhausted. Sometimes just sending a guard out to talk a struggling swimmer into shore avoids the need for a more difficult rescue later.

2. Those at the outer fringes of the swimming crowd may have overextended themselves. Although people in the water naturally tend to help one another, they do not always recognize trouble. "I thought he was just kidding," is a comment often heard, so there may be no other source of aid to a drowning swimmer but the watchful lifeguard.

3. Problem geographical areas, such as rips, inshore holes, or sudden drop-offs, are locations in which many fall prey—particularly children, who find themselves suddenly over their heads from stepping into unexpected deep water. Children are the greatest cause of rescues close to shore. Any visually obstructed area between guard stations, as well as corners hidden by rock outcroppings, should be patrolled periodically. Either a scheduled walking guard or vehicle patrol serves the purpose, as long as the station is manned by more than one guard at a time. Unusual crowd gatherings or special circumstances bear checking out. Warnings can be given verbally when necessary, or signs can be posted requesting swimmers to remain in guarded areas. Obstruction of the guard's vision by sun glare is sufficient reason to move the swimming crowd to an area that is visually preferable. Underwater obstacles such as rocks, drainpipes, and the like should be marked and watched since they can cause a fall that submerges a victim.

4. Gestures for help in the water are generally unmistakable.

5. A swimmer heading shoreward but being submerged by waves hitting the back of his head may be gasping for air. Swimmers in control of themselves look behind when they are warned by the noise of water moving; a person in trouble will disregard everything but getting to the beach.

6. Offshore winds can prove a hazardous tease to those playing with inflated balls, toys, and floats in the water. The floating object is blown just out of reach, tempting the nonswimmer or poor swimmer to chase it into deep water. Most often, children are involved; they tire suddenly, cannot grasp the float which is too slippery, or discover that it will not hold them above water. Sometimes a slow leak or air valve that opens unexpectedly leads to difficulty even in shallow, calm water. These inflated devices create overconfidence in poor swimmers who then venture out of their depth. If the support device is lost, they are unable to return to shore.

7. Attractive hazards such as offshore towers, floats, anchored boats, or midwater shallow reefs entice showoffs and betmakers to attempt swims beyond their capacity. Visitors to beach areas see native residents performing all sorts of athletic feats and want to copy them. If the visitor is not in the same fine physical condition as those who have been working at their sport, he is quickly beyond his skills and in trouble. Diving from high places is the same kind of challenge. The resident knows where this is practical; the visitor does not, and sometimes only luck may prevent injury.

8. Spring is the most difficult time of the year for lifeguards, because the water is still cold and saps human energy very quickly. It is the first

time many swimmers have been in the water since the previous season, and they expect to perform as they did when in peak physical shape. Furthermore, winter beach conditions still exist, characterized by sudden sand bottom drop-offs, uneven ocean floor, and strong rip currents.

9. Remember, when possibly distressed swimmers are under observation, do not "sweat them out." When there is any question whatsoever as to their need for assistance, respond!

USE OF THE RESCUE BUOY, SAND BEACH

It has been found that victims have more confidence in the rescue buoy or tube than any other rescue device used by lifesaving organizations. The support given to a victim by this rescue device signifies to him the end of his drowning sensation, while preventing him from clutching onto his rescuer. Any rescue buoy must be designed so that it (1) is not too bulky to swim with, (2) has a smooth surface, and (3) has no sharp protrusions to injure the victim or guard as they are tumbled into the surf. When making the rescue, the lifeguard notifies his backup team, buckles on his belt or slips into his harness, picks up the can and attached line so he will not trip on them, and carries them with his fins (if needed) as he runs to his point of water entry. A dragging buoy is dead weight, so it is carried until the guard needs his hands to help his forward progress through the water. He holds it also because he wishes to protect nearby swimmers from colliding with his buoy as it bounces through the water.

Since he can run faster than swim to waist deep water, the guard steps with a progressively higher stride as the water deepens, and he keeps his body in a forward position ready to swim. By no means does he permit the water to push him backward. This may involve jumping small waves or diving into larger ones, only to regain a foothold after the wave passes and run again. To gain all possible speed, fins can be used as paddles. The guard holds one in each hand by the fin foot opening and paddles with the blade until he dons the fins to swim. In the absence of fins, the hands are used as paddles while the guard runs, and dug into the sand to pull him forward as he swims through shallow water. He can also grasp handfuls of eel grass or hold onto rock ledges to keep from being washed shoreward as waves pass over him.

The field supervisor may have a buoy that is different in color than those of the rescue team. He is the last person in the water, since his primary function is to direct rescues rather than make them, but his buoy in the water is an indication to the backup team that this job may be a complex one. With his distinctively colored buoy, he can be seen easily and recognized as the man in charge by lifeguard personnel. An example of this special marking would be a two-tone can painted half orange and half yellow.

TAKING ADVANTAGE OF RIPS AND DRAGS

The fastest way through the surf line, of course, is the neck of a rip current. Because a rip flattens the waves as it passes through them and swimming speed is added to its outflow speed, a guard can reach a victim who is caught in the same rip very quickly. Drag caused by long shore current parallel to the beach may move a swimmer rapidly without his knowledge. When he notices, he may panic. The guard takes advantage of the drag to intercept and rescue his victim by simple target tactics. As he runs down the beach planning his entry and swim, he realizes that the same drag will move him. Swimming against it or even maintaining a position is very difficult, and valuable time could be lost. Correct calculations will allow the victim to be carried by the current to the guard as he swims from shore.

THE RESCUE SWIM

The guard should watch the victim as much as possible and should swim with head held high and practice ducking waves and blinking the stinging salt water from his eyes so that he can continually return to visual contact with the victim. This avoids overswimming and missing him. Since the friction of the water will hit the towed buoy with its greatest force after the wave has passed over his body, the guard must learn to expect the extra drag. When ducking waves, the guard should go deep enough so that the rush of water does not push him backwards, yet not so deep that he impedes his own forward progress. In making his rescue, the guard uses all his ability to reach the victim as soon as possible. Some distressed persons will panic but sustain themselves at the surface for considerable time, others will sink rather quickly. The experienced guards will appraise the situation correctly and calmly.

HANDLING THE VICTIM — CONSCIOUS

Guards do not make physical contact with victims unless they appear very weak or about to submerge. He should recover the towed buoy while remaining out of reach of the victim and approach with the buoy between himself and the victim. While extending the buoy to the victim, the guard calms him verbally and tells him to hold onto the buoy. He also watches the victim's eyes for signs of fright and to anticipate any attempt to lunge. Waiting until the victim has gained confidence in both the rescuer and the buoy allows the guard to rest by treading water. The guard should then instruct the victim in grasping the handholds or bridle and ask him to help by kicking as he would when swimming.

If the victim is weak, it will be necessary to stay close to him instead of the usual procedure of towing him behind on the extended buoy line attached to the belt or harness. In this case, the guard often swims in a backstroke position with the victim towed on the buoy just at the guard's side or partially resting on his chest. Any physical contact, such as handholding, is very reassuring to a frightened victim as he is supported only by an impersonal buoy, but be sure that he is calmed sufficiently so that he will not approach you from the rear and grab at you.

During the rest period, explain to the victim that he must not release the buoy in the surf. Despite its light weight on land, the buoy can be a dangerous projectile if it has been pushed underwater and is then driven by a wave out of the victim's hand to be catapulted into the guard's body. In telling the victim what to expect, the guard must observe victim response carefully.

In oncoming waves, a guard may have to hold the victim onto the buoy (if he cannot accomplish this himself) by going to the victim's rear, locking him in, and holding the buoy against the victim's ventral side. The guard must keep one hand free to be placed over a weak victim's mouth and nose if it is necessary to duck under waves. This will prevent him from breathing water. If the guard does not want the waves to push him toward the beach because it may be rocky or undesirable for exit, he must submerge with the victim as the waves pass over. In any case, the victim can be soothed by as much explanation of what will occur as time allows, making sure to advise him to take a breath of air at the proper time.

HANDLING THE VICTIM — UNCONSCIOUS OR SEMICONSCIOUS

Use of the life belt type rubber "tube" buoy designed to snap around the victim's waist enables a guard to float a body with little worry that it will slip out. This buoy is not suitable for very small victims or children if strapping them into a rescue device is required. It has no handholds and must be worn or gripped to be effective. The tube buoy is grasped in the guard's hands, pulled to the victim's chest, and snapped into place so that the line and hook come off at the victim's back. In this way, he can be towed in a face up position and can breathe easily. If for some reason the tube buoy is being grasped instead of worn, the snap hook must be watched so that it does not scratch or cut anyone when driven by rough water.

When using a solid cylinder buoy for an unconscious victim, the device is placed across the victim's chest, as his back is to the guard. The rescuer grasps the buoy by reaching through and under the victim's armpits to prevent his slipping off. With fins, a strong kick will be all the power needed to push both to shore. In an exceptionally large surf, it is wise to swim seaward to calm water until help arrives or until the victim can be swum laterally down the beach to a safer area.

For mouth-to-mouth resuscitation in particular, the tube buoy is most effective because the guard has no worry that the victim will slip away from the supporting buoy. If the victim is not breathing, mouth-to-mouth resuscitation will be required at once as the guard simultaneously moves the victim outside the surf zone. Maintaining this position and the rhythm required for resuscitation is very difficult in heavy surf. Water blown into the mouth, nose, or lungs as a result of wave action can cause pneumonia or other complications. Since you may consume a great deal of energy in resuscitation, swim at a pace that will not exhaust you while working your way to calmer water. If the victim is in a rip, its current will do the work of carrying you seaward. Place your hand under both of the victim's armpits so that you can hold onto the bridle of the can while supporting the victim's upper torso under the backside, leaving your other hand free to aid in resuscitation. If the nonbreathing victim is closer to the beach than to the outside of the surfline, allow waves to push you both shoreward.

Only experience can help the guard in making such precise decisions when the most important consideration is opening an airway that will restore the victim's capacity to breathe. Seemingly, there are more actions required than one person can handle, so the guard's training prepares him with signals for assistance and communication—for example, I need help (upraised arm): victim not breathing (upraised arm waving). At the second signal, a resuscitator can be readied on shore or on the approaching rescue boat, and additional personnel can be ready to respond.

MASS RESCUES

Where many people are in need of help simultaneously in the same general area, the guard in most instances would choose to rescue first those who are in the most serious condition, then those at the farthest fringes of the crowd. As the first guard on the scene attends to the most immediate emergencies, the backup personnel can reach other struggling people.

Unstrapping a buoy and handing it to one victim or a group while the guard swims to others leaves him vulnerable to attack by desperate people. Only as a last resort should a lifeguard part with his rescue buoy. One or more buoys may be taken by the lifeguard responding to a mass rescue. The rescuer should bear in mind, however, that each additional rescue buoy creates considerably more drag in the water. The rescuer may verbally direct troubled swimmers to approach and cling to the safety of the buoys as the guard swims among them and ultimately to shore. The lifeguard may also seek assistance from the stronger swimmers in the area, and the entire party can be encouraged to kick and move to any swimmer who is not able to reach safety.

In the case of mass rescues, no rest period is available to the guard as he readies the first victim for the return tó shore or rescue boat. All possible speed must be used, even in dropping off the first victims in shallow water close to rescue operations where backup personnel can bring them to safety, in order that the rescuing guards can return to other victims.

If, in the confusion, a guard is grabbed by one or more persons, the most effective means of freeing himself is to inhale and submerge. These people are looking for a way to stay above water, and when the guard is no longer supporting them, they will release their hold. Rescuers are more in control of themselves and their breath-holding ability than panicky victims, who will quickly push to the surface for air. The old wive's tale of striking a drowning man is false. There is no way for a rescuer in the grasp of a victim to achieve so strong a blow. Such an attempt is not an acceptable lifeguard technique.

If a victim fights, the guard should stay in a protected position behind him and get a good hold onto his hair or body to prevent him from clutching. Sharp words or angry exclamations can sometimes make the victim or group refrain from moving forward on the buoy line. In a critical situation, it may be necessary to release the harness or belt and swim a short distance away. The buoy will support the victims until the guard can convince them that they must hold it, not him, so that he can continue the rescue.

In white water, only experience can tell a guard what to do. Should a group be distressed suddenly, as in a flash rip, the floating devices of nearby swimmers may be called into action to help support victims, as long as warnings to avoid contact are given to the inexperienced assistants. An effort to assemble victims into groups is the secondary objective of the first lifeguard who reaches the scene of a mass rescue. This grouping should be encouraged only where there are adequate floating devices; otherwise swimmers will hang onto each other, submerging everyone. Although some types of rescue buoys are capable of supporting as many as three cooperative victims, they can handle a few more if the people are small, lightweight, or using it only for rest and not total buoyancy.

SCUBA DIVER RESCUES

Scuba divers in the midst of white water are often dragged down and tumbled because of their heavy equipment. Other times they require help fairly far out to sea. Scuba divers may surface unexpectedly because they are out of compressed air, physically disabled, or badly frightened. Due to the weight of the equipment involved, the larger buoys should be kept on hand in areas frequented by divers. Particular notice should be taken when a diver is looking shoreward without his mouthpiece, snorkel, or mask in place. Circling around to look for a safe exit, swimming to a dangerous place because it offers a handhold, or any extraordinary behavior may be a sign of trouble. Scuba divers are especially attracted to rock beaches because of the abundant sea life there. Therefore, guards in these areas should be given special training in awareness of divers' habits. Loss or damage of equipment may cause the scuba diver to swim with his head out of water, exhausting himself rapidly, or he may be gasping for air in this position, having torn off his faceplate and breathing apparatus to free his mouth and nose. Looking down to drop a weight belt that is submerging him may be a sign of difficulty, as are waves washing over the back of his head or a life vest that has been inflated. All these activities would cause a guard to watch the diver very carefully.

Currently, scuba divers are being trained to inflate vests in order to swim from place to place or rest in the midst of a dive. So while they do bear watching, other signs of distress will probably accompany this symptom if they are in real trouble. Remember, a scuba diver can drown in the shallows where everyone else is safe because he cannot get to his feet as the weight of his gear is no longer supported by water, or because he has become entangled in kelp. Divers are subject to a variety of diseases related to breathing air under pressure. When such a condition seems probable, prepare for backup medical help. Some knowledge of these illnesses, the first aid for them, and the location of a hyperbaric chamber is useful.

Every effort should be made to rescue divers with their gear intact and to discard gear only as a last resort, when retaining it endangers the success of the rescue. At times, just dropping a weight belt or holding out a helping hand may be all the assistance needed. Divers appreciate the lifeguard's concern for their expensive equipment as well as their lives, and good public relations is enforced by safeguarding their gear. An exception is the speargun, which (if cocked) must be disarmed and tossed away to protect both the lifeguard and any nearby swimmers from potential injury.

SURFER RESCUES

Surfers generally have better than average water skills. They have the additional safety factor of a support device—their surfboard. Furthermore, surfers surrounding a distressed victim have boards of their own to assist when help is needed. Guards themselves use boards as rescue devices under certain circumstances (see below). Signs of surfers in difficulty are (1) attempts by novices to power the board by leg strokes rather than paddling in the correct manner, (2) attempts to propel the board sideways, (3) weak paddling, (4) failure to progress through the water because of rip conditions, and (5) continual falling off the board. In general, guards keep a watchful eye on new surfers, particularly if they are in an area that is geographically dangerous for whatever reason.

Most surfing accidents are a result of the surfer being hit by either his own board or someone else's. The victim generally requires medical attention after being brought out of the water. The lacerations are commonly severe enough to need stitches, and broken bones are not unusual. Unconsciousness or disorientation can lead to drowning. Accidents are extremely difficult to detect. The surfer falls in a wave and may not surface. When a guard witnesses a "wipeout" he should try to watch for the surfer to reappear. Any unusual circumstances would initiate a rescue—for example, a surfer holding his head and behaving in a disoriented manner.

Although these athletes are generally in good condition, their knowledge of the sea and their swimming ability may be inadequate once the board is lost. The American Surfing Association, the national amateur governing authority, is stepping up its educational progress, and this will help. However, no guard would ever make the mistake of failing to proceed with a rescue simply because he judged the surfer to be a good swimmer. As a matter of fact, a surfer who is well-known on the beach is at some disadvantage. The guards and his friends are inclined to think that he is skillful enough to handle any situation, disregarding the unpredictability of the sea or the individual's current state of health.

A surfer who has made an easy trip through low waves may suddenly find that he is "locked" outside the surfline when the waves grow larger, and he may be incapable of making the return trip or be too frightened to do so. If a boat or helicopter is available, rescue is simple. If not, the guard will have to swim out after an attempt to communicate by loudspeaker or other available means has been made. The surfer should be encouraged to paddle toward the guard for assistance through the surf. Good surfers are often an attractive hazard to novices, who are tempted to duplicate the board skills of the experts. Using the loudspeaker (if available) to warn obviously inexperienced newcomers may prevent later difficulties. Bellyboards (paipo boards) have many of the same hazards as surfboards and often bring less qualified swimmers to the surfing areas.

FUGITIVE CAPTURE

Certain situations that a guard may face are rare but do occur. One such is the escaped fugitive who enters the water in an attempt to evade the police. The guard should be aware that a weapon may be involved, such as a knife or a gun. Once he has determined that this is not a factor, the lifeguard proceeds as he would toward a hysterical swimmer determined to attack. The guard works behind the swimmer to grasp his clothes or hair and to hold the fugitive submerged if necessary to make capture possible. If there are two guards at the scene, they can alternate in the struggle until the fugitive is unconscious or in need of resuscitation.

ATTEMPTED SUICIDE RESCUES

Suicide can be accomplished by many means in the water. If the victim has attached a weight to himself, there is little hope that the lifeguard can prevent death. Once the victim has jumped from a pier or other high place or swum seaward to the point of exhaustion, the suicide rescue is the same as those described above. The guard must use his experience and intelligence to handle the victim; most often more than one guard is needed to deal with a fighting and/or desperate suicidal individual.

CLIFF AREA RESCUES

High cliffs that descend sharply to shallow water are often scenes of accidents involving people who have fallen or jumped. Any lifeguard station in this kind of location should be equipped with one or more floating stretchers. The stretcher must allow entrapped water to drain rapidly and hold the patient firmly inside. Any stretcher that holds water would obviously become very heavy, since water weighs about seven pounds per gallon, and would add to the rescue hazards. The stretcher may be secured to a flotation device that permits the victim to be floated to safety.

In addition to the normal rescue difficulties, in a cliff accident, victims may be injured or in shock. A patient in shock needs his body temperature kept as near normal as possible—an extremely difficult task in cold water. Covering him with a blanket will help somewhat; although it becomes very heavy as it absorbs water, it reduces the wind's chilling effect. An alternate tool for the guard station without stretchers is a rescue board floated by several guards who protect the two sides or each corner so that the victim will not roll off.

CAR ACCIDENTS IN WATER

The lifeguard service is called regularly to car accidents involving a vehicle that has plunged into the water. If the guard can free dive to the wreck site, sometimes he can effect a rescue at once. If, however, the victim is trapped inside, the rescue is often hopeless. Trapped air inside the car might last long enough for completion of a rescue if the guard can think and act quickly.

Victims of water auto accidents are sometimes able to free themselves and are lying injured and unnoticed nearby. If the guard tosses a small object into the current, its direction may give a clue for the search in areas of moving water. Unfortunately, still ponds and lakes do not offer this opportunity. Inspection of pilings in the location of water bridge accidents, other structures, or nearby points of land may lead to a wounded victim's recovery. Scraps of clothing will sometimes point the way to his route, and the guard's own judgment as to what action he might have taken if involved in this crash, considering the peculiarities of the accident site, is helpful.

Accidents after dark are complicated by the lack of visibility. Assuming that the victim was conscious and seeking escape from the water, what were his choices? Time is, of course, a vital factor in locating the drowning or injured person.

AIRPLANE ACCIDENTS IN WATER

Airplane disasters involving a near-shore water crash or boat sinkings present similar problems. If the guard is nearby and free dives to determine what aid he can give, caution should be used. A faceplate will allow him to see more clearly and explore thoroughly, but at all times sharp-edged, ripped metal and broken glass are to be considered. Aids to finding wreckage include bubbles from the trapped air inside the vehicle, oil or gas leaks, the smell of gas, and floating debris.

FOG RESCUES

Fog often appears unexpectedly in coastal areas and is occasionally associated with the hot weather that attracts large crowds to the beach. As the fog appears on the horizon and begins to move shoreward, the guards should warn the crowd by loudspeaker, advising that the lifeguards will be unable to provide maximum protection and requesting that they move into shallow water. When the beach is finally shrouded in fog, the guard station will issue repeated messages over the public address system to establish a directional beacon for persons still in the deep water. Divers who were underwater and surfers seaward of the surfline, as well as swimmers at a distance, may be able to find their way to shore with the help of this repeated announcement. New arrivals to the beach should be advised of the lack of visual protection available.

A fog patrol by beach vehicles is instituted along the water's edge. Sounds coming from the water (voices, boat engines) can warn the guard that a rescue may be needed. With the help of the patrol, the entire beach is covered in this manner. If a rescue is necessary, one guard enters the water, another radios for a backup crew and gives his location while sounding his horn at regular, short-spaced intervals. When the surf is pounding noisily, sounding a siren will be much more effective than a horn because it can be heard at a greater distance. These sounds from a vehicle at a distress point help the backup unit to find it, as all teams are moving blindly, with only general location instructions. The rescue vehicle should be parked as close as possible to the line of the distress call. When the backup team arrives, the guards space themselves along the beach in the area of the call and in sight of one another, if possible. In very dense fog, the man in charge has to decide how far apart the units of the team can be spaced. At a verbal signal, everyone moves into the water simultaneously. One guard should remain on the beach to sound the horn or siren, so the team members can find their way back.

When the victim is found, the guard shouts to his team so that they can come to his aid or return to shore. If currents have carried the rescue group down the beach, one guard returns to shore and moves the rescue vehicle down the beach, so that the rescue party will intercept it the moment it touches land.

Occasionally an anxious person is discovered wandering on the beach looking for a companion left in the water. He should be picked up and allowed to direct the unit to the point where the missing person was last seen. Clothes left on shore or fresh footprints on deserted sand beaches may be clues. The backup unit is notified.

Calls from normally unguarded beaches follow the same procedure. Guards who cover any part of the shoreline should know their whole jurisdiction in terms of access routes both to and from each beach and rescue routes at those points. A rescue that involves listening and making voice contact with a calling victim forces the guard to keep his head out of the water most of the time. Any guard who is making a search and becomes lost himself can listen for the sounds of the surf indicating shore and can generally assume that the wind is blowing from the open sea toward land, since this is the weather condition that created the fog blanket in the area. The beeping horn or wailing siren of his team will bring him to the rescue vehicle site.

Any miscalculation in navigating boats caught in a sudden fog and attempting to stay in sight of land and find shelter can leave them disabled in the surf or crashing on reefs. Locations near harbor entrances are particularly likely spots for such accidents, and they should be patrolled carefully in the fog. During these special conditions, each beach unit should have an assigned patrol area to avoid duplication and facilitate maximum coverage.

Night calls are generally similar to fog condition calls because of the limited visibility, although landmarks such as street lights, house lights, or neon signs may be useful reference points. Units that make night calls should have one buoy set aside and labeled "night emergency rescue buoy." This tool is equipped with an underwater flashlight. The best type is the plastic rescue buoy with one or more blinker lights molded into it. If this equipment is not available, underwater flashlights should be carried by each swimming guard so that he can be seen in the water, as well as having a light source at hand to help locate the victim.

ROCK RESCUES

Entry and exit from rock beaches present different problems than those of sand beaches, although the rescue techniques are similar. Since the rocks as well as the sea life growing on them can cause considerable injury to a guard, it is important that he start swimming as soon as possible after entering the water.

His procedure for equipping himself with buoy, line belt or harness, and fins has been previously outlined. He will have to

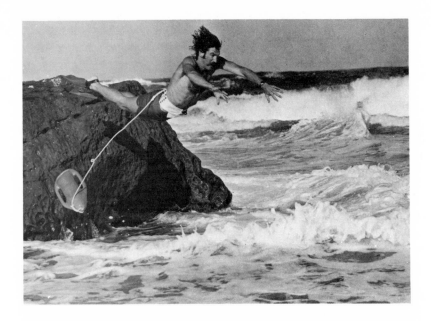

decide for himself at what point he can put on the fins to protect his feet from the rocks but avoid tripping if the blade should bend under his foot as he runs. Running in fins takes practice, and caution must be used where rocks are slippery. When running seaward, take special care to avoid collisions with rocks. The guard should use his hands to help feel his way as soon as possible, while keeping his eyes on the victim. He should swim over the rocks instead of running among them as soon as possible, even though only in knee to waist deep water, and continue to grope with both hands as he swims, holding onto rocks or kelp when a wave hits to avoid being pushed backward.

If entry must be made from a ledge, the guard makes the shallowest dive possible. A bellyflop or racing dive is the most desirable, since any other kind of water entry may take him straight to the rock floor. Although additional time is needed to judge the best moment for entry, it is important that the guard wait for a swell to cushion his fall and not to land in a trough between waves. Confronted with the necessity of making forward progress through oncoming waves, yet wanting to avoid hitting the rocky bottom, the guard will need his good judgment as to how deep to submerge. Ducking under a wave with the head being the last part of the body to submerge is a useful trick that surfers use, and it is preferable under these curcumstances than to a head first surface dive that can lead to head injury.

As always, speed in reaching the victim must be measured against the safety of the guard whose skills are a drowning victim's only chance of survival. Swimming to the victim, calming him, and using the buoy are the same as on sand beaches; however, exit from the water presents some new problems. It may be impossible to remove the victim from the water at the guard's point of entry because of high rocks and crashing surf. The guard should be prepared with an alternate rescue route. It may be necessary to move seaward of the surf and remain there with the victim until the backup unit, boat, or helicopter arrives. A substantial swim to another part of the beach may be necessary in order to exit safely. Any time when heavy surf will assuredly hit lifeguard and victim, the guard should go up to the victim rather than leaving him extended on the tow line and be ready to remove him from the buoy if ducking under waves is required to avoid their full impact.

If the victim has been calmed and prepared for the ordeal in the surf, it will be possible to return to the beach in a relaxed manner. Stiffness and body tension lead to striking bottom or reefs. If rocks are going to be struck inevitably, the guard first uses the buoy as a fending device but finally has no choice other than to allow the victim to hit. Injury to the guard might eliminate any chance of rescue, and both parties could be lost.

There is one advantage in lifeguarding a rock bottom beach, because the shore conditions remain relatively stable. Obstacles in the water, such as holes and current changes, vary little with the seasons even though larger waves and rips customarily accompany winter. Each guard should make a point of studying his beach carefully to note the day's conditions and should remain aware of the changes that take place as the hours pass. Special factors such as sharp corals or dangerous sea life should be studied and prepared for before an emergency arises.

PIER RESCUES

Guarding from a pier has the virtue of quick access to a trouble site by jumping, often very near a victim, and avoiding a hard swim through the surf. Knowledge of water depths at every point around the pier is essential for the guard. If pilings are marked for depth, bear in mind that these figures change with the tides, currents, and seasons.

At all times jump (do not dive) feet first with buoy, line, and fins held over the head at arms length to avoid injury by falling on top of them. Upon hitting the water, if necessary, release the buoy and don your fins. If the victim is not in white water, it is common practice for a guard to toss the buoy to the victim first and then jump to assist him. Use caution, because surf may pull the buoy from the victim's grasp. Drag and wind direction must also be taken into consideration when attempting to throw a buoy near a victim, so that it will be within easy reach but not strike him.

Obviously, another exit must be planned, as the height of the pier makes it useless for rescue unless it is uniquely equipped. A particular difficulty for guards with victims caught under a pier is that they move toward the pilings for support. The sharp-edged mussels and barnacles that grow there can cause painful lacerations, while water movement grates the victim's skin against the rough surface. Try to convince the clinging victim to leave the piling; however, it may be necessary to remove him bodily. If the pilings are going to be hit unavoidably during the course of a rescue, the guard first uses the buoy as a fender, then must allow the victim to take the bumps in order to save both their lives.

Any guard with pier duty should acquaint himself with the side current conditions for the day as he comes on duty and again at the time he initiates a rescue, as he can use this current to his benefit when planning his rescue route.

BOAT RESCUES

Any vessel drifting near the surfline should be watched for signs of imminent distress—the crew working on the engine; people on board waving anxiously to shore; or a position broadside to the prevailing wind, indicating that the boat is either not anchored and helpless or that the anchor is dragging. If the guard takes a bearing on the boat and establishes an imaginary danger line in relation to the surf, he can be quite sure that something is wrong if that line is crossed, even though the bow may still be pointing into the wind.

Disaster can possibly be averted if the guard swims to the boat and offers to tow it seaward by means of a line tied to the boat cleat. A single man can swim and make forward progress with a boat of lengths up to about thirty feet, depending on the size and shape of the vessel and the wind and tide velocity. In practice, several guards would normally do this job as a team because of the implicit danger of capsize and mass rescue. Even if they accomplish nothing more, the rescue team dragging at the end of a boat line acts as a sea anchor and prevents the boat's drift into the surf until a rescue boat arrives. Under no circumstances should any guard swim up to the lee (shoreward) side of a boat. A disabled vessel may overturn at any moment, pushed by wind and waves, and the guard would be in a very vulnerable position.

One of the first things that rescuers do when approaching a boat is to request that all lifesaving gear be placed on deck or even better, worn by the crew so that they are prepared to jump upon command if necessary. If the engine is running, but cannot move the vessel to safety, a swimming guard directs the passengers to shut it off. If a sailboat, the sails are to be dropped and anything that is dragging but not anchoring the boat is pulled up. A slipping anchor may impede rescuers in moving the boat.

Once outside the surfline, the boat's position is maintained until the arrival of a rescue boat. Whatever the means of towing the distressed vessel away from the surf, be certain that it is far enough out to sea so as not be blown into white water before it is underway. If the boat is going to enter the surfline and this cannot be prevented, direct the people on board to jump off to seaward as your team prepares to make the rescues. Should the boat swamp and overturn from wave action, the passengers will not be struck by it if they evacuate on the windward side.

If the boat is in shallow water, several guards or volunteers under their direction may hold it in a bow to sea position so that it can be towed through the surf and to a safe location by means of a line swum to a rescue boat. This is possible only in small surf and favorable winds.

Always be mindful that any aid administered to a boat is given only after the permission of the captain or boat owner has been granted. If the boat captain or owner will not accept assistance, the lifeguard should advise the crew as to the consequences and instruct them to use their life jackets.

Any guarded beach where boats commonly pass should be equipped to handle disabled craft. Some boats have no towline, so a line brought by the guard attached to a buoy with a snap hook that can be secured to any eyebolt on board may be very useful. If the removal of the vessel from the beach is impossible, remove all loose items and equipment to a safe location for the owner to pick up at a later date.

SIGNALS

Because of the difficulty in communicating at sea, signals should be established to permit messages to pass among rescuers and those on land or in rescue vehicles. Some examples are:

1. Raised arm—swimming guard needs assistance.
2. Waving arm—victim is in need of resuscitation, prepare the resuscitator.
3. Rescue buoy raised vertically over beach guard's head—rescue help is on the way (usually backup team man).

4. Buoy raised horizontally over beach guard's head—move victim to a position outside the surfline and wait for assistance (boat, helicopter).
5. When PA systems are absent or muffled by large surf or calling distance is too great, a lightweight, waterproof walkie-talkie worn by the swimming guard permits him to be directed to a victim by spotters and to communicate with his backup.

USE OF SWIM FINS

With only minimum swimming ability, a person aided by swim fins can be an adequate to good swimmer. They allow one to swim strongly without an arm stroke, as they do the whole job of propulsion. They can be compared to the thrust of a motor; they give speed and strength, push through the waves easily, and protect feet on rocky ground. For rock shore areas and pier rescues the guard dons his fins as soon as he hits the water. For sandy beach rescues, the fins are carried during the run to the point of entry and then used as paddles—one in each hand—until the guard is in chest deep water.

Since fins take time to put on, the good guard must evaluate their desirability for a given rescue. If the victim is very close to shore, perhaps at the dropoff, and requires only a few swimming strokes for contact, then the fins are of little use. However, depending upon the tide, size of surf, and slope of ocean floor, improved swimming speed more than compensates for the time used to put on the fins.

Only experimentation can determine the proper size fins for the individual guard. When the fin blade is too large, the legs can become tired and cramp easily. The flexibility of the blade is also a matter of preference. The best style of fin is debatable, but the fit must be correct and the construction must include a solid heel strap. Adjustable straps work loose too easily in the surf, and a fin may be lost at a crucial time. Any type of shoe fin is unacceptable for the lifeguard because the water enters the shoe and pushes on the flat surface near the arch causing the fin to fall off or be pushed off by the pressure of the water. The fin designed with a curved blade is also unsatisfactory because the water rolls off the curvature in such a way that a powerful swimming stroke is impossible. All guards should have fins, and each should be sure that he always wears his own—the ones that he chose to fit his feet and swimming style.

RESCUE BELTS AND HARNESSES

Rescue belts are preferable to harnesses for rock beach rescues, for landline rescues, and for very busy guard stations where a guard may wear his gear all day, carrying his can buoy with him, ready to go. Belts have the advantage of fitting snugly and staying in place during severe ocean conditions. Each guard has his own belt, adjusted to fit him, and his numbered buoy attached, Rescues involving victims laden with heavy scuba gear work much more smoothly with a belt than a harness. The belt is most often adjusted for size by means of a shoelace arrangement that is tightened or loosened to fit the guard's waist. It allows the dragging line to pull along the center axis of the body rather than on one shoulder as with a harness. The belt's width makes it comfortable and keeps it from cutting into the waist when tugged. Since it snaps into place, the guard can hook the belt as he runs toward the water, keeping his eyes on the victim. Picking up the wrong belt by accident can create a problem since either it will not fasten at all or it will slip and impede the rescue.

The harness has its own advantages, since it slips on more quickly than a belt, and one size fits everyone. It is more efficient when the guard has to make many short rescues. Both the belt and the harness should be made of nonrotting material such as dacron, nylon, or polypropylene.

THE LANDLINE

The reel and its coiled landline are a nearly outdated rescue device used prior to the rescue helicopter and boat and in situations where such rescue vehicles are not part of lifeguard equipment or are occupied elsewhere. The main disadvantages of the landline are: (1) It ties up a group of guards when others on the beach may need attention. The only alternative is to select volunteers, who in their eagerness to help often do more harm than good. (2) Landline rescues are time consuming and may not get assistance to victims quickly enough.

This rescue device consists of a reel on which the 500 to 900 feet of line is stored. The reel may be portable or attached to the front or rear of an emergency vehicle for quick transport to trouble spots. When installed on a vehicle, the landline and reel should be easily detachable in case the vehicle is suddenly needed elsewhere during the rescue emergency. A hand-carried portable reel holds less line because of weight restrictions since it often must be moved speedily. All guard personnel should be advised of the length of each landline. Actually, this information should be posted on the equipment so that no guard attempts a rescue requiring 900 feet of line with a rig that holds only 500 feet.

The reel is not to be used for cranking victims and guards to shore. The weight of two or more bodies in the water is greater than that of the reel, making it too unstable to crank. Although the vehicle reel is attached to a heavy base, the handle is generally detachable, making it impractical for cranking in victims.

The correct use of the landline is to bring to shore victims who have been caught in the neck of a rip when the best exit for rescue is against this outflowing water. In mass rescues, a landline facilitates returning to shore with multiple victims.

The method for using this equipment is quite simple. A guard swims to the victim and determines that the landline is needed to complete the rescue. Upon his signal to the backup team, a second guard takes the line. The line is snapped to a buoy by means of a safety clip after being wound several times around the bridle. The hook is not the only means of attachment, since the winding reinforces the connection and removes strain from the bridle. The belt from the buoy is fastened around the guard's waist, and he holds a coil of about seventy-five feet of line in his hand, unwound from the reel, so that he experiences no uncoiling drag as he makes his running start. The line is uncoiled by the shore team at a rate that permits no backlash yet minimizes the drag on the swimming guard. Whenever possible, the reel and shore team are placed at a high point (for example, cliff above the rescue site), since the greater the elevation of the reel, the less the line drags, as it is held by water weight and current.

When the backup guard reaches the rescuing guard, who is supporting the victim, the line guard unsnaps his belt and hooks it to the rescue buoy belonging to the guard helping the victim. Unless there is some reason why more than one guard must support the victim, the second guard can simply hold the line and be towed to shore. There is no point in tiring himself by swimming against the current to move himself out of it when his energies are needed for rescues later in the day. After the victim is safely grasping the buoy attached to the landline, he and the guards are slowly pulled in by the shore team. One guard stays near the victim so that he will not be pulled underwater if the towing is too rapid. If insufficient guards are on hand, bystanders may be used for the towing process, but this practice is discouraged unless essential. If it is a necessity, try to choose young men who are known to the guard group.

In response to prearranged hand signals by the rescuing guard, the beach team speeds up, slows down, or stops the pulling actions through the shifting water. Pulling should be hand over hand in a slow, steady manner that permits slackening for the suction that precedes each oncoming wave. With the slack, the group in the water can go over the top of a wave instead of being drawn into its plunging fall. Sample hand signals are (1) go—wave arm; (2) stop—stiff arm.

The only advantage of the landline is its capacity to bring swimmers to shore through the neck of a rip or against wave action where there is no other possible exit or rescue device. When volunteers must be used, the experienced guard in charge assumes complete command of the operation and demands instant compliance from his amateur crew.

Materials for the Reel

Although wood is sometimes used for reels, it is subject to rotting, and the expansion and contraction caused from sea water penetration loosens its structure. Noncorrosive, lightweight, tubular metal is best—aluminum or steel. Electric reels have proven unsatisfactory, since they corrode in the sea air and they cannot be controlled sufficiently in the stop-and-go circumstances of the landline rescue.

Materials for the Line

The landline should be colored for easy visibility (e.g., yellow), capable of flotation, and of a diameter large enough that it will not cut the hands of rescuers but small enough so that an adequate amount can be wound on a reel. Standard size is three-eighths inch, although five-sixteenth inch is sometimes used. Nylon line used in a storage bag can be colored but it does not float. After the rescue, the line should be rewound on the reel neatly and washed in fresh water at the first opportunity. The only reason for line washing is to remove residue sand, which acts like small knives among the fibers, breaking them down and weakening the line, so it is not necessary to wash the line until a quiet time when there is no chance that it will be needed. An auxiliary line is handy for use during the period when the newly washed line is drying. All lines should be inspected regularly for possible breakage.

RESCUE VESSEL PROCEDURES

The rescue boats are an integral part of the ocean beach lifeguard operation. The rescue boat may be called to back up the beach lifeguard when the beach guard has a long rescue outside the surfline or a riptide with several people being swept out to sea. The rescue boat will swing in to pick up the people and move them to a safe portion of the beach or keep them on board until the surf subsides.

On very busy days, the rescue boat works close to shore just outside the surfline to keep an eye on large groups of bathers and to stand by off the end of large rip currents. In some remote or overcrowded beach areas where land units are severely restricted, rescue vessels may be the only means of transporting rescue personnel to a beach emergency.

The rescue vessels may be called in to assist in medical evacuation from vessels in the vicinity of the beach where the rescue vessel is stationed. The lifeguard vessel also may be called to assist in search and rescue work, downed aircraft, diving accidents, overturned vessels, boat fires, and other related emergencies, including a wide variety of law enforcement functions.

The rescue vessel and crews are called in on resuscitation and first aid cases in such inaccessible areas as cliff bases, breakwaters, and small islands. The rescue boat crews can swim in and give quick attention to injured persons until they can be evacuated by helicopter or other means.

Other Routines of the Rescue Vessel

Rescue vessels and crews, depending on their need or demand, work a variety of daily schedules; however they should be available for call twenty-four hours a day. The rescue vessels may be called (any time of day or night) to pull grounded vessels off the beach, although it is most important to get the people off safely. The rescue boat's crew may have to make quick patches, plug holes, and pump water from the stricken vessels.

When to Call a Rescue Boat

1. The beach lifeguard should call for the rescue boat any time he thinks it can assist him in effecting a rescue or preventing anticipated accidents from occurring in his assigned area.
2. Normally, the rescue boat can give ample assistance in long rip tide rescues or in conditions when the surf is too large or heavy to bring a victim back to the beach. The boat is usually of no use on short rescues inside the surfline because it is too large and heavy to maneuver inside the breakers.
3. The rescue boat should check or investigate the following conditions:
   a. Long distance or channel swimmers;
   b. Life rafts, powerboats, sailboats, rowboats, surfmats, paddleboards, or surfboards manned by the public in distress offshore;
   c. Large floating debris such as pilings, poles, and timbers drifting ashore into a swimming area or causing a navigational hazard;
   d. Powerboats of any class or size that are on or near the surfline or less than 200 yards offshore; or
   e. Any other unidentifiable floating objects, such as dead bodies or the appearance of dorsal fins (whales, sharks, porpoise) in or near a swimming area.

Boats in Distress

The following situations should be investigated to determine if the boat is in distress:

1. Powerboats (any class or size)
   a. On or near the surfline (especially those broadside to the wind);
   b. Trying to start engine, drifting toward surfline;
   c. Rowing any powerboat;
   d. Capsized boats;
   e. Waving arms, clothes, oars, and flags from boats;
   f. Anchored, working on engine over an extended period of time; or
   g. Boats emitting excessive smoke.
2. Sailboats
   a. On or near the surfline;
   b. With broken mast;
   c. Overturned;
   d. Near surfline, tacking back and forth without making headway;
   e. With one or more sails dragging in the water; or
   f. Uncontrolled sails flapping in the wind.

Distress Signals Used by Small Craft at Sea

1. A gun or other explosive signal fired at regular short intervals;
2. A rocket or flare fired at short intervals;
3. Continuous sounding with any whistle, horn, or fog signal device;
4. Flying the National Ensign upside down; or
5. Flying the code flag "November-Charlie."

Reporting Distressed Vessels

Obtain all information possible before reporting to the dispatcher. Try to obtain the following information:

1. Type of vessel in distress (i.e., cabin cruiser, outboard, inboard-outboard);
2. Bow numbers or registration numbers;
3. Identifying structural colors and design of the vessel;
4. Length;
5. Number of persons aboard;
6. Type of distress; and
7. Location (if possible get a line of sight over two or more fixed objects or landmarks to determine the position of the distressed vessel).

This distress information should be as accurate as possible to help the rescue boat crew find the distressed vessel and make preparations for the rescue work. If a vessel is in the surfline, the beach units should advise all persons on board to put on life jackets and prepare to exit the vessel on the seaward side. If time permits they can be advised to make an attempt to anchor the vessel.

What To Do When the Rescue Boat Arrives

1. The lifeguard must obey the commands given by the boat personnel. The velocity of the wind and drift, the height of the swells, and the set of the current determine the proper time and place to haul both guard and victim aboard the boat. Arm signals by the boat crew will help determine which direction to swim out of the rip tide to come to the boat or to return to shore.
2. The guard always approaches the boat swimming with his head up to be able to see arm signals or hear the orders given over the engine exhaust noise.
3. The guard will be told to bring the victim to the step on the stern of the boat. Bring the victim to within six feet of the stern of the boat and stop. Await orders before coming any closer.
4. When it is time to put the victim aboard, the guard should stay between him and the boat until relieved of the victim by boat personnel.
5. The propellers are in constant motion even though the boat has no headway or sternway. Therefore, the guard must be extremely careful not to let rescue gear, his extremities, or those of the victim get underneath the boat.
6. After being relieved of the victim or victims by the boat crew, the beach guard will swim ashore to his assigned station. If the pickup is made a considerable distance from his station, he will be taken to a point directly off his assigned station and dropped off just outside the surfline.
7. The victim will remain aboard the boat to be either taken ashore by the crew at a safer spot along the beach or returned to a docking facility.

How to Make a Rescue from the Rescue Boat

The lifeguard making a rescue from the boat will never, under any circumstances, leave the boat until told by the operator where and when to leave. When given the go ahead signal, the guard should always jump or dive from the stern of the rescue boat and be sure his rescue gear does not become tangled in any of the deck fittings as he leaps into the water.

After making the rescue, the guard should return with the victim either to the boat or, if conditions are favorable, to the beach. If returning to the rescue boat, he should not board until given a hand signal from the skipper that it is safe to do so.

Lifeguard Rescue Vessels with Divers

Very often rescue vessels are called by dive boats to assist with various kinds of diving accidents. When the rescue vessel approaches within of one hundred yards of the dive boat, the rescue vessel crew should ask the operator of the dive boat if it is clear to approach his vessel. When—and only when—given the OK from the dive boat, the rescue boat should approach very slowly and with caution, always keeping a lookout for scuba bubbles. After recovering and transferring the victim, if all the divers are not aboard the dive boat, the same caution should be used until clear of the diving crew area.

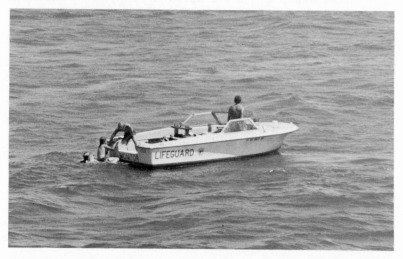

Lifeguard rescue vessels carry members of the dive recovery team on drills and recovery dives. The safest way to work with the dive team is to anchor near the dive location. After the rescue vessel is anchored, the dive flag should be raised, and the divers should leave the boat from the stern, one at a time. As the last diver leaves, the time and depth should be recorded. The propellers should not be engaged until all the divers are back on deck. The divers should remove their fins before climbing back on board the rescue vessel. If scuba tanks are taken off, they should be properly stored so as not to roll.

At some dive locations, the vessel will not be able to anchor. If the rescue vessel cannot anchor by the dive location, the divers again should leave the vessel from the stern one at a time, but all the divers should stay on the surface until the vessel moves away from the dive area. Again, the time and depth should be recorded and the dive flag raised. The rescue boat should stay away from the dive area until all the divers have surfaced. If two divers surface before the others, have them swim out toward the rescue vessel for the pickup.

On some occasions, it becomes necessary to pick up divers from the surfline in order to save time. For a safe pickup in the surf, the rescue vessel backs in near the surf and stands by. The divers should swim out to the boat, one man at a time. Each diver should swim with his head up and toward the side of the stern to avoid being hit by the boat if it lurches back on a swell. The boat crew will direct the diver to the swim step when it is safe and help him aboard. Once aboard, the diver should be seated to allow the skipper to see the next diver swimming out.

Rescue Vessel and Helicopters

When working with helicopters, the rescue vessel's crew should follow all instructions from the pilot. On some occasions, the helicopter will set down on the water. A water landing will take place only if the surface is reasonably smooth. On the water, the helicopter's rotors will continue to rotate. The rescue vessel should avoid coming in close to the rotors on the top or on the tail. Also, the rescue vessel's wake should be kept down so as not to push water into the open hatch on the starboard side of the helicopter.

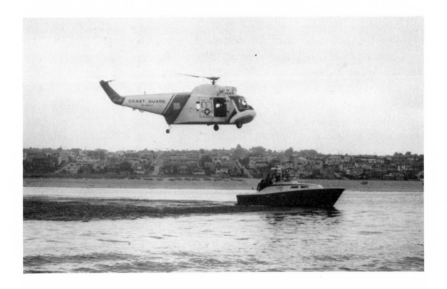

In most cases, the helicopter will drop a cable with a basket attached to pick up injured or disabled persons. To prepare the vessel for helicopter assistance:

1. Lower masts and booms;
2. Pick up loose gear;
3. Provide a clear area, preferably on the stern;
4. Keep unnecessary personnel out of the way;
5. When the helicopter arrives in the area, change course so as to place the wind 30 degrees off the port bow and continue at idle speed;

6. Prepare to accept all required equipment, as provided by helicopter;
7. Allow the basket to touch the vessel prior to handling it;
8. If the basket has to be moved to the patient, unhook it from the hoist cable;
9. Do not move the basket with the hoist cable still attached;
10. Upon removal of the hoist cable, do not attach cables to any part of the vessel;
11. Attempt radio contact with helicopter at once, if possible;
12. Stand by for further instructions.

Approaching Distressed Vessels and Aircraft

Lifeguard rescue vessels are built with a stern step or swim step and a door in the transom. The rescue vessels are built this way to allow the boat crew to work with overturned, disabled, and sinking vessels. The lifeguard rescue boat in almost all cases works with its stern to all types of rescues.

When approaching a drifting and disabled vessel, the rescue vessel should approach the bow of the distressed boat with the stern of the rescue vessel. Stern to bow will enable the boat crew to pass the tow line without the two vessels blowing together.

When the disabled vessel is at anchor, the rescue vessel cannot back in with its stern because of the outstretched anchorline. With the anchored vessel, it is necessary to approach off the side of the bow and move forward with the vessel as the anchor is pulled up.

Swamped or sinking vessels should be approached from downwind to avoid blowing over or into the distressed vessel. The stern should be put in close to the stern of the distressed vessel to take passengers off the boat and put pumping equipment and patching equipment on board. When working demasted or overturned sailboats, the rescue vessel must approach with caution, keeping a lookout for rigging, sails, and sheets floating near the vessel.

If the rescue vessel is called to a downed aircraft, the rescue vessel should use caution if the aircraft is in shallow water. Wingtips might be bent up close to the surface or the tail might be high enough to strike the bottom of the rescue vessel. If the aircraft is floating and passengers are exiting, the rescue vessel should put the stern into the wing to pick up people, keeping a lookout for bent flaps, landing gear, and other debris. If the floating aircraft is military, and the pilot is unconscious, the rescue crew should look for the yellow tags on the safety pins that should be placed in the ejection mechanism before the pilot is removed. If the pins are not in place, the pilot and the rescuer can be injured if the ejection seat is accidently set off. All the pins are tagged with yellow markers and printed with instructions for correct insertion to disarm the ejection seat.

The Surf Rescue Board

The surf rescue board is a lifesaving tool that fits somewhere between a rescue buoy or tube and a surf rescue boat in application. A rescue board will give the lifeguard the flexibility of covering a specific distance in a relatively shorter period of time with less physical exhaustion than if the rescuer swam the same distance. Of course, a surf rescue boat could cover the same distance much quicker than in either case. In a rescue situation where *response time* is very critical, the use of rescue board could make the difference between success or failure over a swimming rescue attempt.

A rescue board does have its limitations. Large surf size and short wave frequency can significantly limit or neutralize the rescue board's effectiveness. The successful use of a rescue board also depends on the user's skill levels.

If the possibility exists that the board could be lost to the environment during a rescue attempt, it is a good idea to take along a rescue buoy or tube and a pair of fins. These can be worn while paddling a rescue board with little interference. If the board is lost, then rescue equipment is still available to complete the job.

The basic techniques for utilizing a surf rescue board are explained as follows beginning with the most elementary position.

Prone

When lying prone, leg position is an important factor in maintaining board balance and preventing rails from tipping or digging" (causing an inexperienced person to roll off). Legs spread toward the rails counter tipping and maintain control, acting as balancing outriggers or sailboat "trapezes." If the board begins to tip, perhaps from a boat wake or wave wash, a leg extended in the opposite direction will counterweight and correct the angle. When the water is very calm or the guard is sufficiently experienced, he will probably be more comfortable with his legs held together and straight or crossed at the ankles. To make minor balance adjustments, a slight roll of the body or leaning of the hips in the direction opposite the tip will counterweight. Oversteering should be avoided. Basic advantages of the prone position are that (1) it is a stable, resting attitude; (2) it offers little wind resistance, slowing wind drift and giving added control when hit by a condition such as "rotor wash" from a helicopter; (3) turning is executed easily by sculling with hands, as explained for the sitting position. One disadvantage is that the prone position limits visibility to water level sightings unless the trunk is continually lifted in a modified "push-up."

Motion is achieved by extending the hands into the water alongside the rails and paddling. The action should begin with both arms entering the water as far forward of the guard's body as possible. The arms are then drawn down and back with the limbs fairly straight and the hands cupped, cutting deep into the water in something like a "butterfly" swimming stroke. The stroke is repeated rhythmically with quick, smooth thrusts as in rowing a racing shell. An alternate stroke when arms tire is an arm over arm "Australian crawl" movement. The thrusts remain quick, smooth, and rhythmic. This second stroke is less tiring but does not give the acceleration or power of the butterfly. To maneuver the board while paddling, drag the arm that faces the direction desired and scull with the other hand and arm; for a slow turn, simply pull harder with one arm than the other.

Kneeling

The guard kneels on both knees at the center of the board maintaining equal balance on all sides. Knees should be spread comfortably but no wider than shoulder width. Body weight is distributed by sitting on the ankles or calves with arms at the sides, hands gripping the rails, and weight on the palms. Hands can also be placed on knees or thighs. Of the many variations of this basic position, the guard will choose the one that suits him best. He may balance on his knees and arms, thus supporting his chest, shoulders, and head. Hands will grasp the rails with weight on the palms. Counterbalancing is achieved by shifting body weight to the knee opposite the tipped rail and extending the arm on that side. For acute rail tip, the hand on the tipped rail can pull up, while the guard's body weight is pushed down on the opposite hand and knee. Too much force applied too quickly will cause the board to flip over. To turn when kneeling, the guard sculls the water with his hands. The heightened visibility is a distinct advantage of using the rescue board in this position, although the high center of gravity lessens control somewhat. Wind resistance is considerable and affects board drift, while fatigue is often experienced in the knee area from the pressure of prolonged kneeling.

The paddling position while kneeling begins with arms extended as far forward as balance allows with the body bent at the waist and the upper chest, head, and neck almost parallel to the deck. Keeping the center of gravity low for control and balance, the guard uses the butterfly stroke, pulling as deeply through the water as possible, striving for power and speed. For added speed, the upper body weight can be rocked downward before each stroke, forcing the board to sink slightly. As the stroke begins, the board will be pushed back up from the water it displaced in the rocking motion. Correctly timed, this upward motion can be directed forward so the board moves forward as it is paddled. In knee paddling, the body weight is shifted a little further back than when kneeling on a stationary board. The tail block will ride lower than before, but with a forward motion the block will plane on the water, causing it to rise, which forces the nose down. A disadvantage of knee paddling and the high center of gravity is the difficulty of maintaining a victim aboard, while advantages include power, speed, visual height, and generally, less fatigue.

Sitting

The guard sits astride the board deck, and usually faces forward with a hand on each rail, on his hips, or wherever comfortable. With his body at the center of the board, balanced so that he is level in the water, the guard can shift his weight to achieve a nose-high or tail-high position as circumstances direct. Counterweighting is accomplished by extending an arm, leaning the body, or "pushing" from one side at the water with a single kick, out and away from the rail opposite the tipped side. Turning a stationary board in this position can be achieved by

1. Sculling-rotating each foot and lower leg toward the desired direction, one after the other in a synchronized manner, so that the feet meet each other at the inboard rotation and are furthest apart at the outboard part of the rotation; and
2. Tail block pivot—a shift of the body weight to a point about half-way back from the balance point of the board. At the moment the nose of the board starts up from the shift in weight, the guard leans back and well toward the direction of the turn simultaneously extending the arm opposite of the direction of the turn outward and holding a rail well forward of his body position. Simultaneously, the guard leans back pulling the rail with a jerk toward the turn direction. At the same time, the guard kicks hard with both feet and legs, causing the board to pivot around the sunken tail block. With experience, one man can turn the board almost 360 degrees with a single hard kick, a strong continuous pull of his arm, and the body weight thrown into the turn with spirit. The secret of the tail block pivot is aggressiveness.

The sitting position offers the advantage of high visual plane and little fatigue for long periods of time. A disadvantage is great wind resistance, which causes drift. An effective way to offset drift from mild winds or sometimes strong currents is to point the board in the direction of the wind and/or current and rhythmically rotate the lower legs at the knee. If the left leg is rotated counterclockwise and the right leg clockwise, giving considerable thrust to the rear of each rotation (using the remainder of the rotation as a recovery part of the stroke to position both legs for another backward thrust) the body can be left free to aid forward motion at the moment of thrust. The pelvis is pushed forward at this moment in a seesaw, rocking movement. These combined actions will maintain a board in a near-stable location when landmarks are being lined up to locate a victim or during a search and recovery operation.

METHODS FOR LAUNCHING

Still Water

To achieve a good, fast launch under these optimum conditions, the initial glide is maintained as long as possible before commencing to paddle. On sand beaches the guard can gain good speed by running with the board, with the bow pointed toward the water. The guard must run until he is in about knee deep water or until he reaches the dropoff. When the appropriate depth is reached, the guard grabs the board by each rail at about the center, deck inward, and without letting go he "throws" the board at the surface of the water. When this motion is followed by the momentum of his own weight, the board is propelled at considerable speed for a short distance like a stone skipped over the water. When the board hits the water, the guard throws himself onto the deck and assumes either the prone or kneeling position in the same manner as one would in starting a snow sled down a hill. As the board's glide speed slows, the guard begins to paddle. When the victim is twenty to thirty feet from shore, the guard can launch and glide to the victim without paddling. To avoid hitting a victim, the board is aimed at a point clear of the body. The same launch, without the run, can be used with success from a low dock, reef, rocks, platform, or the like when the water is at least knee deep. Without the run, however, the glide is significantly shortened.

Launching in the Surf

Experience and skill are assets in maintaining forward progress through the waves, never allowing them to push the board toward shore. The guard uses the same aggressive running launch as on the sand beach until depth and oncoming water force him to begin paddling. In other words, he starts paddling at a point where he can no longer run as fast as he can paddle. In most cases he can outrun the in-rushing water, except perhaps, in very small surf. Advantages should be taken of any lull between sets of waves, and launches from low heights should be timed to hit the back of the last wave of a set where the water is deepest. If a backwash is moving off reefs, rocks, or a steep beach, the guard can time the launch to get a boost toward open sea. On rocky or reef-filled beaches, one would seek an entry that does not receive the full brunt of the surf. Areas with sharp dropoffs between rocks or deep holes where waves re-form permit a faster and easier launch than fighting shallow bottom waves.

Launching in Shallow Water

Where a long, shallow shelf must be traversed before deep water is reached, as at low tide, running with the board may be fastest over a smooth sand bottom; but if the bottom is pitted with holes, rocks, or other obstacles that restrict running, the board may be launched in even fin deep water and paddled with a shallow stroke. If the water is shallower than fin depth but still deeper than the board is thick, the guard can turn the board wrong side up, providing the rocker isn't too great to restrict passage. He can paddle prone or knee paddle or pull the board along by hanging onto kelp or rocks. Since so many shallow water beaches have strong currents, advantage should be taken of any current that will move him out to sea to a spot where he can paddle faster. If, conversely, the current will move the guard too far from the rescue site, he must compensate by entering the water at an appropriate distance up current. A good launch provides instant acceleration and a significant glide, which quickly reduces the distance between shore and the victim and establishes a safety margin between the paddling guard and the hazardous shore environment. This margin is especially crucial when bad conditions could force a rescuer back onto the beach before he can achieve a paddling "head of steam."

METHODS OF MEETING AND CROSSING WAVES

Frequently, a guard must fight his way through the waves with great determination in order to reach a victim. For success he must combine all his physical skills and practical experience. When use of a rescue board is impossible, it is the direct responsibility of the guard to make a correct judgment before the rescue is attempted, and only the trial and error knowledge of his training can aid his decision.

Small waves up to three and a half feet or so can be passed simply by lifting the rescue board, laying it on top of the wave, and allowing it to support the guard's prone weight. Once established, the forward momentum of the board will be maintained as the waves roll underneath. A board can "sled" through the water as the guard is running, instead of being carried in about waist deep water. The board is pushed along at either middeck, midrails, or tail block; in the first two positions it is easily controlled over or through small, oncoming waves. Just before the full force of a wave hits, the guard can swing his body onto the deck and take an off center prone position, or he can lift his body high over the rails with his arms and let his legs trail back with the passing wave. Once the wave passes, the guard can regain his footing and proceed.

Pushing Through

"Pushing through" means exactly that when meeting the power of an oncoming wave without leaving the ground or losing balance. When waves are breaking with significant force, a guard must have enough forward momentum to offset the shoreward force. Waves must be approached at right angles, and the moment of break avoided, if possible. For sufficient momentum, the guard must paddle especially fast and strongly prior to wave contact; this is probably accomplished best in the prone or kneeling position. Just before meeting the wave, the guard grabs both rails and lunges, throwing his body weight forward to keep the nose of the board down. If his weight is not forward, the wave will lift the nose and force the board up and back. In pushing through small waves with relatively little force (up to two to three feet), the guard can approach the wave in nearly the same manner, with the nose only a little higher than for normal paddling. At impact, the guard grabs the rails and raises his body in a push-up manner off the deck, allowing the force of the wave to pass between his body and the board. The prone position offers more control for most people than the kneeling position, with less chance of losing the board. However, the knee position lets the guard see what is beyond the wave that is about to hit him, and while continuing keep visual contact with the victim.

"Rolling" the Waves

A technique used to escape the force of a large wave is to turn the board over, allowing the wave to pass. When trying to pass medium to large waves, a guard will find that by rolling, he will suffer considerably less abuse than by pushing through. In effect, he is attempting to match or surpass the collision forces of a wave, a feat that may be possible for small waves but not when dealing with tons of pressure from large ones. When a life is to be saved, the guard must "bend like a stalk of grain or break" under colossal water power and must allow it to roll over him as he exerts a minimum of forward momentum. Just before the impact of the oncoming breaker the guard inhales deeply and flips over with his board while holding the rails close to its nose. In this situation, the fin is up, and he is underneath.

Taking advantage of his forward momentum and the downward curve of the rocker, the guard holds on tightly and forces himself and the nose of the board as a single, bonded unit as deeply as possible underneath the force of the wave. At impact, the guard forcibly holds the nose down and jerks the board underwater to expedite the duration of the roll and to offset the circular upward pull of the surrounding water. Once through the wave, the guard rights himself and continues paddling to the victim. If any of the wave's force hits underneath the board's nose, the board is pulled away from the guard. If the guard maintains his grip, he would be forced with the board up and "over the falls"—the breaking face of the wave.

The main sensation of rolling in a big wave is that the wave is trying to suck the board up and away. This sucking effect is countered by jerking the board underneath the breaker, pulling down hard at the nose and trying to keep body weight bonded to the board. In some cases, wrapping the legs around the board helps to retain possession. Occasionally this sucking or lifting action can be used to advantage in smaller waves, as the guard can let the wave start to take the board and then jerk the nose through the back of the wave at the proper moment, causing the wave to release it prematurely. At that moment the board and guard will shoot up and out from the momentum caused by the lifting water freeing them.

In spite of these techniques, guards should make every effort to avoid surf while using a rescue board. They should enter the water during lulls and ride through the waves on rips in order to take advantage of their "deep water effect." Naturally, bottom configuration, position of the victim and his condition, wave conditions, and surrounding environment (rocks, reefs, sand, and the like) play a major role in the final judgment as to when, where, and how to reach the victim.

In extremely large surf a guard may wear his rescue buoy and fins while paddling out on a rescue board. Then if the board is lost or abandoned, he is not left without rescue aids. Only with rescues that do not involve heavily congested swimming crowds, such as those during winter months or at locations not within the usual range of guard stations, would these complex techniques be attempted.

METHODS FOR PICKING UP A VICTIM

Conscious victims should be approached with caution, as in any type of rescue. The guard should make the nose of the board available to the victim for support, but at any sign of panic or aggression by the victim, the guard should dismount on the side away from the victim, leaving the board between them. Now the guard is in control of things and a safe distance from an irrational person. Verbally the rescuer can calm the victim, instruct him to mount the board, and describe the course of action that will take them safely to the beach. The victim, once reassured and more confident, can think of something besides his present precarious plight.

For very weak, semiconscious, or unconscious victims, the board is maneuvered alongside and behind the body. The guard immediately lifts and supports the victim's head and shoulders onto the board, face up. Simultaneously, the guard dismounts on the opposite side, using his own weight to counterbalance that of the victim. If the victim is not breathing, the head is cocked back to straighten the windpipe and open an air way. Mouth-to-mouth resuscitation is begun at once, followed by the rescuer's signal to the beach or rescue boat for assistance and to ready a resuscitator. All the guard's efforts should now be directed toward sustaining the life of the victim and moving him away from surf or any other dangers. He would make no effort to return to shore with this victim, but would wait for assistance.

If the victim is strong and able to help himself, the guard can simply instruct him to mount the deck of the board facing the nose. Once the victim's head and shoulders are supported by the board, the guard can aid him by pulling his legs onto the deck. The victim is instructed to keep his head and body down in order to maintain a low center of gravity.

If the victim is not strong enough to mount the board, the guard proceeds as follows: (1) The board is dismounted and turned upside down between the victim and the guard so that they face opposite rails. (2) The guard reaches over the bottom of the board and grasps the victim by both wrists, pulling his arms across the board until the rail is next to the victim's chest and under his armpits. (3) Holding both overlapping wrists with one hand and grabbing the opposite rail with the other hand, the guard bobs up out of the water with a strong kick and, as he comes down forces his body weight down on the near rail. In the same motion the guard pulls up on the opposite rail until the board flips over and lies deck up supporting the victim's upper body. The guard then swings the victim's legs into place, finishing with victim flat on the board, head forward.

If the victim is a scuba diver, water conditions must be considered before any gear is removed and before he is placed onto the board. With a reasonably strong victim and good water conditions, the gear-laden victim in need of support can be assisted onto the board. When conditions are bad or the victim is weak, first attempt to get assistance before removing his gear. Although it is quite easy to transfer a tank and weight belt to a can buoy, if one is available, if time or conditions do not permit this, "ditch" the gear and raise the victim onto the board.

By grasping the victim's legs just below the knees, the guard can push him forward on the board, or by the ankles, to the rear, to adjust for trim, correct nose angle, and to prevent purling. The guard can accomplish these adjustments at any time, when he is on the board or off, but the victim should be warned to prevent panic or sudden compensating movements on his part. Weight adjustments are a bit more difficult during scuba diver rescues since the victim is heavy and thus causes the board to ride deeper in the water than usual. The guard must be in constant control of the trim as well as the "rail dip" caused by the high center of gravity of the diver's tank.

METHODS OF MOVING A RESCUE BOARD WITH A VICTIM ABOARD

In most circumstances, once the victim is on the board and his weight has been adjusted to also accept the guard's weight, the guard is ready to paddle them both to safety. The guard takes a prone position over the victim's hind quarters with the victim's legs on either side, adjusts the trim, and starts to paddle. Although the kneeling position can be used, it is less stable than the prone attitude. Since the full weight of the kneeling guard is supported by the board, unless the victim is very small and light or the board is unusually buoyant, it will ride with the rails underwater. Forward progress with a sunken board is slow, tiresome, and unstable; in short, the prone position is much easier on the guard and on the victim. To expedite the rescue, a recovering victim can be instructed to assist by paddling, and there is little chance that he will slip off if controlled by the prone guard.

When a victim cannot be paddled to shore, the board is used as a floating platform to support the victim as he is towed to shore by the swimming guard. Examples include very weak victims or heavily laden ones when the weight of the guard added to the weight of the victim would submerge the board. The most stable rescue technique has the guard control the board by counterbalancing from the tail block. An injured victim who cannot support the prone guard over his hind quarters or maintain board balance (due to a fractured or dislocated arm, leg, hip, or collar bone, for example, or severe lacerations) can be swum to shore by a guard pushing from the tail block and using a scissors or frog kick. A guard who realizes in advance that he will have to swim the victim and board to shore would take his fins on the rescue as they do not interfere with paddling. When two victims are in need of rescue, a guard who considers conditions safe and the rescues feasible may place both on the board and swim them to shore. However, this should be attempted only if no other assistance is available; it would be much wiser to wait for help while supporting the victims outside the white water.

MASS RESCUE TECHNIQUES USING A RESCUE BOARD

The rescue board can provide an effective life support means for a mass of victims who need buoyancy until they can be moved individually by guards to shore or a nearby rescue boat. The first guard to respond to this kind of emergency can take his board and fins as well as one or more can buoys to offer maximum assistance until the backup crew arrives.

RETURNING TO THE BEACH WITH THE VICTIM(S)

Although it is possible for a guard to bring one or more victims to shore through surf using a rescue board, it is a gamble. Even in small waves, the slightest misjudgment or tip could cause the board to broach or purl, turning a routine rescue into an emergency. In lieu of bringing the victim through the surf, the guard should remain in calm water with the victim until transferred to a can buoy, boat, or helicopter. If he has no other recourse, the guard proceeds to shore with extreme caution. The guard should avoid attempts to catch or ride waves with victims aboard; this feat may be dramatic, but it only invites trouble. Instead, slack periods of water movement between waves should be used as much as possible. When caught inside by a wave, the guard should shift all the weight to the back of the board. Holding the victim, the guard tells him to maintain a good grasp on the board until the wave passes. The guard can even sit on the tail block and hold the victim's legs or lie prone on top of the victim, forcing his body weight down on the hind quarters beneath and grasping the rails tightly. The guard can also dismount, pull the victim toward the tail, and hold both rails as he straddles the victim with his chest and arms holding him secure with body weight.

These are all methods for offsetting the disrupting wave force. After each wave passes, the guard can resume his shoreward progress while keeping an eye on the waves behind. Once the guard and victim are well inside the larger surf, where loss of the board would cause no more harm than embarassment, small waves can be used to aid the progress to shore. Purling and broaching are best avoided when riding waves by keeping weight well to the rear of the board and using the feet and hands from a prone position to stabilize the board. Again, gatherings of bathers are to be avoided.

Bringing a victim to shore in still water is quite simple and self-explanatory. The only obvious problems are deciding the best landing site and avoiding hazards, obstructions, and swimming crowds. Awareness of prevailing currents, rips, kelp, menacing rock formations, or floating debris will ensure successful rescue efforts.

Victims too weak to stand should be walked through the shallow water lying on the board and pushed by the guard. As the guard reaches the shallows and sees that the victim will not be able to walk under his own power, he dismounts, tells the victim to lay prone or places him so, adjusts the weight to trim the board, and pushes the board nose first. If he is walking in surf, he keeps his body perpendicular to the waves as he walks and does not permit waves to hit the board broadside. If for some reason the board is parallel to an oncoming wave, the guard never permits either the victim or himself to be in its path, as serious injury could result. To retrieve a loose board that is moving sideways, the guard should attempt to grab the nose or fin and tail block from the side, swinging the board around until it is perpendicular to the surf. If the surf is still large enough at walking depths to hamper moving the victim to shore, the guard can turn the board nose to sea and let the shoreward wash help to bring it in as he controls it. The nose should be kept high enough so that water will not wash over the deck and hit, choke, or upset the victim.

USING THE RESCUE BOARD AS A STRETCHER

Because of its design, the rescue board can be substituted for a stretcher when necessary to bring a victim out of the water and up on the beach. With the victim centered properly, guards at the nose and at the tail can lift and carry the board. As an extra precaution, a guard at either side of the victim will prevent him from falling off, because a board carried in this way tips readily. Progress should be slow and deliberate if possible.

CARDIO-PULMONARY RESUSCITATION ON A RESCUE BOARD

With at least two operators, cardio-pulmonary resuscitation can be performed on a rescue board as long as it is in calm water. The victim should be laid across the width of the board, face up; his chest is the area that requires the most support. This position stretches the throat and gives the victim a natural airway. One guard, stationed at the victim's head, keeps the airway out of the water and administers mouth-to-mouth resuscitation. The second guard straddles the board and faces the victim's chest to apply heart compressions. In cases where the heart is beating but the victim is not breathing, mouth-to-mouth resuscitation can be applied in the straddle position by a single rescuer.

COORDINATED HELICOPTER RESCUE

Of all the forms of transportation available to lifeguard services, the helicopter is the fastest, most agile, and versatile. Many lifeguard agencies around the world are currently utilizing the helicopter as an effective lifeguarding tool. Since there are many different types of "choppers," some of the following information will not be applicable to all of them. The lifeguard agency will have to coordinate area needs, financial resources, and desired tasks to be performed with available aircraft.

Many municipalities develop a working agreement between their lifeguard service and another branch of local government that operates helicopters. These agreements result in having a chopper on standby for the lifeguards on all big or rough surf days. In most cases these agencies provide one of their helicopters as a transportation and rescue vehicle.

The most obvious usage of the "chopper" is to transport the guard, with his rescue buoy, to the scene of a water rescue. Upon arrival at the scene, the lifeguard exits the helicopter and effects the rescue. Then he will either swim to shore with the victim or return to the helicopter.

In order to incorporate the superior transportation functions of agency-sponsored helicopters, and with the need to transport emergency lifeguard rescue personnel, training sessions are conducted to familiarize lifeguard personnel with the pickup techniques of rescue helicopters. Helicopters of the Coast Guard or other sponsoring agency usually not only have the capacity to fly greater distances and, as fuel is consumed, to haul sizeable payloads but also may have to be able to land on water. When sea conditions are suitable, the crew may choose to land the helicopter in the water, using a metal ramp to allow lifeguard personnel to actually swim and then climb into the helicopter from the starboard side. While this method is very quick and efficient and could allow fully equipped divers to gain immediate access to the helicopter, sea conditions often prevent such a landing.

When landing is unreasonable, the power winch from the helicopter may be used with different baskets styles either to lift lifeguard personnel and/or victims into a helicopter for transport or to lower necessary equipment onto rescue boats or into the water. Basket hoists are a bit slower than the landing technique, but are easily managed, particularly in light to moderate winds. The accompanying photographs show transport of a fully equipped scuba diver.

For a fuller understanding of helicopter rescue operations, it is necessary to discuss each method in greater detail so that rescue personnel may fully appreciate this type of transportation.

Basket Transport

A number of conditions must be met for the helicopter to safely transport personnel or equipment to or from surface craft. First, the helicopter is quite unstable unless it is moving ahead or is headed into a relatively mild to moderate wind. In order to stabilize the helicopter, the pilot would fly above a forward-moving rescue vessel at approximately five miles per hour. While this speed is not critical, it can be improved by an understanding of the combination of wind velocity and movement of surface craft to enable a ten-to fifteen-mile an hour current to pass over the helicopter rotors. Logic would explain further that the surface craft should be headed, for the most part, into the wind as the helicopter flies overhead. Helicopter pilots normally hover above the surface craft so that the pilot can have a clear view from his starboard side down to the vessel to coordinate the speed and direction. The surface craft should keep the wind thirty degrees off the bow on the port side. This enables the helicopter to head into the wind for best maneuverability.

Helicopters for Use in Searching Open Seas

Many times, it is necessary for lifeguard agencies to coordinate open ocean searches that come to their attention through radio communications calls. In such cases, the helicopter is quite superior not only for covering vast areas of open sea but for its superior vantage point, with its altitude giving a very broad view of the open ocean. From that view you can also see between swells and chop that might otherwise obstruct the vision of search groups on surface craft. In addition to searching a broad segment of open ocean, the helicopter can also be used to look for submerged objects such as boats or drowned victims. When lighting conditions are favorable, the use of polarizing sunglasses helps to reduce surface reflection and makes it possible to see below the water surface if the actual clarity of the water permits. It has been very helpful to use Coast Guard helicopters for viewing platforms, particularly when someone or something is known to be submerged in an area. Such aerial surveillance should be kept to reasonable periods of time in which a life may be saved or a quick recovery made of whatever it is that is lost, as currents will undoubtedly move the drowned victim or even a boat over time. It is excessively expensive and unnecessary to use helicopters over prolonged periods in submersion searches.

Aerial Search with Searchlights

In addition to the U.S. Coast Guard, many other local government agencies have helicopters available, particularly police and fire departments. These helicopters are frequently equipped with high intensity search lights that are of tremendous benefit in nighttime searches of restricted areas of potential water accidents. These lights are of various types and capabilities and should be investigated by lifeguard agencies prior to use. Some high intensity lights are rigidly mounted on the helicopter flight path, but the width of the beam may be adjusted in accordance with the altitude of the helicopter during the search. The higher the flight pattern, the more the beam of light must be restricted, to create suitable intensity for illumination at the surface.

However, since non–Coast Guard helicopters are not equipped for water landings, restrictions may be placed on using them extensively over water. If such a restriction exists, it may be advantageous for the shoreline beach lifeguard services to arrange funding for suitable pontoons for at least one of the aircraft. Such arrangements are quite suitable, particularly on those rare occasions when a helicopter is needed for rescue in close proximity of the ocean surface. Such pontoon-equipped helicopters would not be encouraged to land on the ocean surface; rather, the pontoons ensured safety in the event of mechanical failure of the helicopter.

Helicopter Platform for Coordination of Surfline Rescues

When surf conditions are particularly adverse, rescues from surfline areas may become so time-consuming that it is impractical for shoreline guards to return to the beach with victims. In these cases, most agencies would tend to accumulate their victims on board the rescue boats, which eventually will become overcrowded and unable to respond suitably and quickly enough to further rescue activity. Here the helicopter can provide a long-range view of oncoming swell patterns, communicating with surface craft and directing the rescue boat when and approximately where to make shoreline runs to ferry accumulated victims into quiet water during lull periods.

Another job for the helicopter crewmen is to manipulate winch controls for lowering the basket to the rescue vessel. A danger is created at this point by the static electricity built up by the helicopter motor as it passes through the atmosphere. Such static electricity will discharge on the first contact with a person, surface craft, or water and can be both very alarming and dangerous unless they are understood and expected. In order to create a partial discharge without hazard, an insulated boat hook should be used, or at least lifeguard personnel can slap at the stretcher or basket to provide a partial discharge before actually grabbing it and guiding it onto the rescue boat. Once this contact is made, there is no further concern for this discharge as the winch cable will continually ground it to the boat and into the ocean water. If it becomes necessary to leave the basket on board the boat for a long period of loading or unloading, it is vital that the stretcher not be secured to the rescue boat until the winch cable has been unhooked and separated. Helicopters must have the freedom to move according to changing wind currents and cannot in any way be secured to substantial surface craft. The winch cable hooks are extremely easy to operate and should simply be unhooked and hauled away until it is time for the helicopter to retrieve the basket and its contents. Helicopters may also transport additional pumps or medical aid supplies to rescue vessels using the same method as transporting a person in the stretcher.

Basket Pickup of Personnel in the Water

When it is necessary to pick up rescue personnel or victims from the ocean, the basket will be lowered as the helicopter hovers fairly close to the surface. It is advisable to allow the basket to enter the water to fully discharge the static electricity before any physical contact is made by rescue personnel. Once the basket is in the water, the floats will support it in a mostly submerged position, allowing lifeguards to enter it for emergency transport. Hand signals can be used to give necessary directions to the helicopter crew. Voice communication from the surface to a helicopter is practically impossible because of the excessive noise of the helicopter engines and rotors. In such basket pickup operations, it is necessary to be aware of the tail rotor and to counsel anyone else in the water with you near the rescue scene to stay well away so as not to inhibit the movement of the helicopter in any way. As air currents may change suddenly, it is unlikely but still possible for the tail section of the helicopter to dip severely, which could allow the tail to injure anyone in the vicinity.

Only one person at a time should be hoisted on the basket winch cables. Overloading the winch system would provide an unstable condition for the helicopter and could cause an uncontrolled crash into the ocean. Another concern, particularly to the rescuer, is water being splashed by the prop wash, which if continually looked into would probably severely hamper vision. The rescuer needs to keep his head averted until vision is specifically required to load the basket and signal its hoisting. When being hoisted into the helicopter, it is vital to remain in the basket entirely: No arms, legs, or equipment must be permitted to extend beyond the confines of the stretcher or basket. It is also important to remain stable in the basket until the crewman in control of the winch system gives directions to the contrary.

Ramp Pickups

As earlier mentioned, if surface conditions of water and wind are suitable, it is highly advantageous for the helicopter to land and load using an extended ramp. In this case, a metal grading is suspended from the starboard side of the helicopter with support cables, allowing the crewman to step onto the ramp to give physical assistance to lifeguards or victims being unloaded. Again, static electricity is of some concern, and to assist in its discharge, the crewman will use a metal pole (a boat hook, for example) to discharge the electricity and to assist the approaching personnel. Of tremendous concern here is the need to have an open and clear area within which the helicopter can manipulate the tail section. The tail rotor in a landed situation is rather close to the water and there would be tragic results if anyone were struck by it. The ramp pickup is otherwise the most efficient means to quickly take on one or more individuals.

Helicopter Use Near Cliffs and Beaches

In mild to moderate wind and weather conditions, helicopter use adjacent to a cliff is possible but complex. However where cliffs are abrupt and vertical, terminating in deeper water, it is nearly impossible for a helicopter to approach the cliff base for any kind of pickup operation. Unless the cliff is a relatively low one, the helicopter is also unable to stabilize itself above the cliff, as the basket cable is limited to one hundred feet. A further problem of operating around a cliff is the erratic and turbulent action of winds near the cliffs, which may be compounded by helicopter rotor wash. When conditions adverse to the helicopter use develop, lifeguard agencies must resort to another rescue form.

There are not many problems for the helicopter landing and picking up personnel or victims off a sandy shoreline beyond that of curious beach visitors coming close to the helicopter to see what's going on. Lifeguard agencies must maintain the strictest crowd control measures possible to eliminate any possibility of a beach patron being struck or hindering a helicopter rescue operation. It is of special concern to the helicopter crew that sand not blow into the operating mechanisms. In mild wind conditions, this is apparently not too great a problem, but if wind developing conditions are carrying sand, dirt, and dust in a horizontal movement, it becomes necessary to wet down the area by means of helicopter rotor wash. Helicopters approaching a potential landing area almost always circle the area first to develop a feel for the wind as well as to survey the surrounding obstacles, not only for the immediate landing itself, but for the potential of being disrupted in liftoff by changing wind conditions. Were changing winds to affect the aircraft, the pilot must have a suitable operating area in which to take off in a more horizontal manner, as opposed to a vertical lift.

Physical Requirements for Air Flow

For helicopter flight, the rotors must be capable of either biting into new air or compressing the air beneath them against something of a solid nature—either land mass, a building, or water. When operating over the ocean, swell conditions should not have a tremendous influence on the stability of the air mass under the helicopter rotors when hovering, but the surface winds that frequently accompany swell conditions will have an effect on the helicopter. It is helpful for the air mass to be moving horizontally so that the helicopter rotors can bite into new air, but when that air flow becomes erratic or becomes quite strong, the pilot must continuously compensate in order to maintain a fairly fixed position over a rescue or pickup site. While helicopters have the ability to hover, each helicopter according to its size has a varying capacity depending on payload and air densities. Air densities at sea level are fairly stable, particularly in the ocean environment, enabling the helicopter to hover quite consistently.

Wind conditions for helicopter flights in the vicinity of shoreline cliffs, as previously mentioned, are quite erratic, so that helicopters require suitable operating space to facilitate maneuverability as well as flight to leave the area. Increased wind velocities cause a turbulence than can adversely affect helicopter use, so lifeguard services should be prepared to resort to alternate means for rescue operations, particularly in close proximity to cliff areas. Lifeguard services should also be prepared to expedite alternate means of rescue by surface craft whenever wind and visibility and general weather conditions do not permit the safe and effective use of helicopters, even over the open ocean.

For all practical purposes, helicopter flight depends on the feel and visual senses of the pilot. If, as in adverse weather conditions, he does not have the horizon or stable structures to judge the altitude of his helicopter, it may be very difficult—if not hazardous—to proceed. The same holds true for flying in turbulent air. By the time the air has influenced the helicopter and the helicopter makes an abrupt movement, the pilot must again be able to relate that movement to his lifting or landing chore. When such turbulence is repetitive nature and intense, it may be hazardous for the pilot to attempt to use the helicopter in close proximity of other persons. One additional note of consideration for rescue work in the vicinity of a cliff area is that if it is possible for a pickup zone to be located at the top of the cliff, it is most desirable for the pilot if that pickup zone be near the edge so that he can approach in an up-wind overland landing pattern. After landing or pickup, the most acceptable short liftoff is to take the helicopter over the edge of the cliff and "fall off" —so to speak—to accelerate and get the rudders into a maximum of new air for the escape flight.

Helicopter Towing of Surface Vessels

While it is true that the helicopter has a significant towing capability, such towing must be done only under the most desirable conditions and only with the full understanding and control of the helicopter pilot. As mentioned earlier in the chapter, securing a helicopter to anything very substantial can cause the pilot to lose control, particularly if gusty winds of adverse velocity were to strike the helicopter from a unknown or unexpected direction. It is therefore important that lifeguard personnel on a vessel requiring assistance be certain that any towing be attempted only after full and thoroughly understood communication with the pilot. For example, in a panicky situation, if the pilot were to come overhead and lower a cable or a basket, some unknowing, unsuspecting person on board might secure that cable on a towing bit or such, expecting to be immediately towed to safety. This could happen even if lifeguard personnel on board knew that this is not the intention. It is therefore an absolute requirement that lifeguards be most definite in their understanding and communication with the helicopter crew if any kind of towing or heavy lifting is to be attempted.

Communication Between Surface Craft and Helicopters

It should be pointed out that helicopters use their unit number when making radio calls. This number is painted on both sides of the jet intake just above the pilot. It is also a great help to have lifeguard rescue boats identified by number on the top deck for easy identification from the air.

CALM WATER LIFEGUARDING

First and foremost, the supervisor, manager, or head lifeguard must assume the responsibility of learning all he can about the history, origin, and topography of the body or bodies of water under his supervision. The reason for this is obvious; he must be aware of the types of recreational use planned for the area and prepare to have hazards marked or publicized to the public using it. Most inland waterways provide boating, fishing, water skiing, and most importantly, swimming. With these things in mind, the supervisor must be aware of the following:

Natural Topography

By knowing the history of a given water area, the supervisor can acquaint himself with the type of bottom and other natural conditions. A manmade body of water (usually the result of a dam) will present the greatest challenge to the lifeguard. Inland waterways will normally have a fine mud silt bottom with near-zero visibility. It will be fed by local drainage and be stirred by wind and other disturbances. A natural lake may tend to have a rock and sand bottom with vegetation. This allows good visibility and its own type of hazards. Under ideal conditions, where you have sand and a rather strong stream of water entering or leaving the area, you should look for quicksand conditions. Around the mud or silt, the dried top crust is easily broken through as is ice on a frozen lake. The mud can cause panic and fear as the victim becomes trapped. There may be holes or severe slopes (shore or beach) leading into the water and continuing below the surface. The hazards of the inland lake can be numerous and varied. By becoming familiar with these hazards, the supervisor can impart this knowledge to the public and the staff. One important fact is that the water level and its fluctuation should be controlled to prevent flooding. If not, what provisions are made for removal of equipment and personnel in case of flooding?

Lifeguard Training

As mentioned above, the supervisor, among his many duties must impart his knowledge of the area to his lifeguard staff. History, topography, normal skills of lifesaving, and knowledge of first aid, defined swimming, fishing, and boating areas are all a part of the training.

The lifeguard may operate from several different positions or pieces of equipment—shore patrol, walking in a designated swim area, sitting in a lifeguard tower, paddleboard patrol of a swim area, rowboat (flat bottom boat), or powerboat patrol away from the swim area.

A rescue buoy (float) is a lifeguard's first piece of equipment and must be with him at all times. Multiple rescues by one lifeguard are not uncommon in calm water.

Still water, warm water, and lack of distance perception are just three dangers to the swimmer in a roped swim area. Warm water will keep the swimmer in the water longer. Lack of wave action and the appearance of a nearby buoy line can lead the swimmer to go beyond his capability. When he becomes tired, the lifeguard must be alert to the rescue.

Use of the rowboat and paddleboard speak for themselves. The training of lifeguards using these two pieces of equipment should include proper turning techniques and methods of pulling victims onto or into the boat without turning over. The lifeguard must keep his distance from the swimmers and discourage them from "hanging on" and talking.

Debris

An area where fishing is allowed can, unfortunately, lead to a condition of general debris from fish hooks, broken bottles, and other hazardous articles. A bottle patrol is always a good practice prior to opening of the swim area, because sharp objects in a calm water area (as opposed to a surf area) will stay sharp. Rocks, submerged limbs from trees, vegetation, and mud (silt) bottoms present added problems in the shallow part of the swim area. It should be noted that often when a person sinks into silt, a cut from any item can result. For example, a tin can resting on the bottom can be covered with layers of silt. If a victim sinks in the mud to his knees, he could sustain a serious cut from this hidden can. Efforts should always be made to dig out such debris. A few minutes with a rake each day can often provide a relatively debris-free swim beach and wading area.

Powerboat Training

The lifeguard who operates a power boat must be made aware of the piece of equipment entrusted to him. Loss of control of the boat can cost the swimmer a limb or his life, as can allowing swimmers to get too close to the propeller. The wake of the vessel, if not properly controlled, can cause injury or personal damage to fishermen, water skiers, and other persons. The powerboat lifeguard has many duties and responsibilities. He must patrol the entire water area and have a complete knowledge of submerged objects such as vegetation, rocks, shallows, trees, and deep channels. He is an extension of the shorebound lifeguard. He must have full equipment to handle any shoreside emergency—namely, rescue buoy, complete first aid kit, resuscitator, anchor and line, oars, radio (communications), fire extinguishers, and where possible, a small paddleboard to reach very shallow areas. On a large inland waterway, two lifeguards should always be on the patrol boat, because one must operate the boat in an emergency while the other (deckhand) can go over the side for a rescue or throw a line to a disabled boat. Most states have inland boating laws. The supervisor and patrol boat lifeguard should know and apply the local laws to his lake operation.

Swim Area and Shoreline

The swim area is the heart of the calm water operation. Swimmers will range from one or two individuals to a large group.

Choice of the swim area depends on the type of location. The ideal swim beach is a very gradual sloping beach with no submerged objects or debris. It has a sand or gravel bottom with good clarity and maximum sun exposure. Where there is a mud bottom, attempts should be made to import sand for the beach as far out into the swim area as possible. Buoy lines can be incorporated where necessary to insure adequate separation of swimmers and persons engaged in other types of activities such as boating, water skiing, and fishing and to provide adequate safety precautions. The distance at which buoy lines are set will depend on depth of the swim area, number of users, and availability of lifeguard personnel and rescue equipment.

Avoid lines that run from shore to outer limit of swim area. This can be a great contributor to drowning, as the nonswimmer will go hand over hand into water over his head.

Posted signs are often overlooked and become part of the landscape to the public. Signs used should be within your facility area to point out the location of your swim area—and no more.

Shoreline Precautions

Swimmers in an unauthorized area are almost unavoidable on large lakes. No wading should be permitted. No swimming outside the designated area should be permitted. Consistent patrols and enforcement of regulations are an absolute must!

Fishermen

Do not allow any fish hooks in the swim area or overhead casting in a populated area. This also applies to fishermen in boats. They should be kept away from the swimming area at all times, day or night. The fisherman has the entire area; the swimmer does not.

Boating

Local boating laws should be adhered to at all times. The average safety perimeter around a swim area can run from 200 to 300 feet. This is vital to the safety of the swimmers. Water skiing is best confined to an area away from swimmers and shore fishermen. Where possible, use a cove or the lake center (where the lake is large enough) with provisions made for shore takeoff and landings for skiers. All ski boats should have two occupants. One operates the boat, watching at all times in front of him. The other is the ski observer watching the skier. The observer notifies the operator when the skier being towed falls or wishes to be dropped off on shore. The observer has the responsibility of notifying other boaters trailing behind a downed skier. This is best done by raising a brightly colored flag (international orange) contrasting to the water and shore.

Pleasure Boaters

On large waterways, sudden wind storms can topple boaters into the water and blow them away from their boat. There are many types of boating accidents. The lifeguard should always be in a position to effect a rescue of an overturned boat. If he is on shore and sees a boating accident, he should be equipped with a rescue board or make attempts to notify his patrol boat via radio if possible. As a last resort, he should swim to aid the victims with his rescue float.

Non-water-skiing boaters should not be permitted into the water ski area, while ski boats should be confined to it. Again, try to organize your water area according to how large it is, the size of the boats permitted, the horsepower of the engines, and—most important—speed limit.

The size of the body of water dictates what types of activity can be permitted and in which areas. Local boating laws must always be adhered to. Above all, life jackets are the most important item in any boat, and should be worn by the boater.

Additional Hazards

Lakes, bays, and other inland bodies of water usually have poor or nonexistent surface water visibility. This is mostly due to plankton blooms or disturbance to the bottom, which mixes bottom sediment into the water body. Poor or nonexistent visibility hides underwater hazards, which should be marked by buoys or warning signs. Many serious accidents occur when persons dive or jump into dirty water hiding such hazards as submerged rocks, pilings, trees, and other similar objects. Sometimes persons dive or jump into shallow water they think is deep, with serious injury resulting. Two other hazards that lifeguards assigned to poor water visibility areas should be made aware of follow.

1. Storm drain pipes that deposit drainage onto sand beaches create a potentially dangerous situation. The sand in front of them will wash away, leaving large depressions that extend well out into the water. These depressions many times exceed the average height of people and cover a large area. Unaware persons wading can step immediately over their heads when walking parallel to the shoreline in the vicinity of the pipe deposit area.
2. Most lakes and bays have drop-off areas underwater where waders can unexpectedly step over their heads. These drop offs are usually parallel to the shore line and run its length. This is especially true of manmade or altered bodies of water.

CLIFF RESCUES

Cliff rescues involve highly specialized rescue techniques that involve diligent practice to perfect. There are four common methods to remove a person who is stranded on the face of a coastal cliff or bluff. They are the (1) descent control device ("sky genie"), (2) stake line, (3) the Mechanical Advantage System (M.A.), and (4) the mechanical crane unit.

Descent Control Device

The rapid descent control device is better known by the trade name of the sky genie. The device, which can be used by one man, operates strictly on the principle of friction created by turning a nylon line around an aluminum shaft. The device allows a single man to get to the victim of a cliff accident safely and quickly.

The maximum speed of descent depends on the number of times the nylon line is turned around the shaft. The number of turns is determined not only by the lifeguard's desired rate of descent but also by his body weight. For example:

1. Extremely Rapid Descent. Two turns for the first 150–200 pounds, one additional turn for each additional 50 pounds.
2. Fairly Rapid Descent. Three turns for the first 150–200 pounds, one additional turn for each additional 50 pounds.

When using the device in wet or humid conditions, removing a half a turn compensates for the added friction caused by the swelling nylon rope. It should be noted that the "sky genie" has a minimum safety factor of 2500 pounds, and its soft, braided nylon, five-eights inch rope has a test strength of 3000 pounds. The length of the line should be sufficiently long for the steepest cliffs in the areas where it is to be used.

Other equipment that is needed along with the actual descent control device is:

1. A belt with adjustable back and seat straps, with an oval locking snap-ring;
2. Two iron stakes, suggested minimum size two and a half by two and a half by three-sixteenths inches and three feet long;
3. A sledgehammer;
4. A safety helmet with chin strap for each man, and safety goggles (minimum of two); and
5. A lightweight back pack.

The lifeguards should drive the stakes into solid ground near the top of the cliff if there is no other suitable place or object to secure a

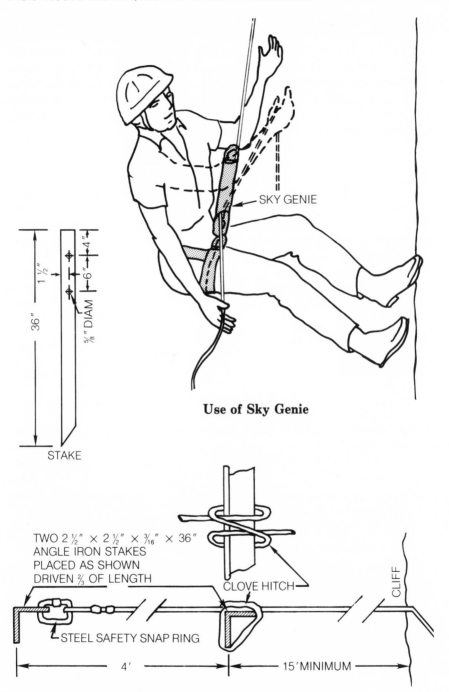

Use of Sky Genie

Lines and Stakes at Top of Cliff

line. Then the lifeguard can attach the descent control device and make sure it is functioning properly prior to descent. For example, the locknut on the shaft of the sky genie should always be checked to make sure it is secure. The guard will then descend to the victim and upon reaching the victim, will reassure the person that all is under control. The victim is placed so his right leg is over the guards left hip and his left leg is over the guards right hip. He will be facing the guard. The guard then completes the descent, pausing as necessary to maintain proper balance of the victim. If a lifeguard is lowering himself down the face of a cliff to assist someone at the bottom, the descent can be made more swiftly than with a victim.

The descent control device should be checked following each use to insure cleanliness before storage. The rope should be checked for cuts or abrasions and to determine if it has dried out. If the rope becomes soiled, it can be washed like any synthetic material in a mild detergent and hung to dry. The line should be stored in a chain stitch manner, starting with the end away from the snap-ring, to help eliminate tangling.

Mechanical Advantage System (M.A.)

The M.A. System is used to provide greater lifting power than could be provided by direct pull. The increase power is theoretically three to one but friction will reduce the actual advantage to about two and a half to one. An M.A. System can be set up in either a vertical or horizontal plane.

1. Equipment Required
   a. Two rescue pulleys (substitute four carabiners),
   b. One anchor sling (three- or six-inch nylon webbing),
   c. Two Prusik slings (9-mm blue perlon line), and
   d. One adjustable sling (three- or six-inch nylon webbing).
2. Component Parts of System
   a. Anchor. The anchor must be absolutely and unquestionably solid. Locate anchor as close to fall line above victim as possible and above level or working surface.
   b. Anchor Sling. Use three- or six-inch nylon webbing. Anchor sling should be as short as possible and still maintain working room.
   c. Anchor Pulley. Two aluminum rescue pulleys are carried in the hardware pack. If no pulley is available, use two reversed carabiners. Clip pulley into locking carabiner and then clip to anchor sling. Pulley must not rest on ground or be forced against rocks. This could jam the pulley and or increase the frictional force.
   d. Traveling Pulley. Take pulley and clip to traveling Prusik with locking carabiner.
   e. Anchor Prusik. Use 9-mm blue perlon line to tie Prusik knot. Anchor Prusik may be attached to the same point, as anchor pulley.
   f. Traveling Prusik. Use 9-mm perlon line.

Mechanical Crane Unit

The third and most effective method for making cliff rescues is the use of an electrically controlled crane mounted on a cliff rescue vehicle. The total boom reach of such a unit should extend at least to twenty-two feet in order to avoid parking too close to the edge of a cliff. A lifeguard using such a unit should never operate the boom at any time within six feet of any high tension lines or stand under the boom. The unit's wheels should always be checked before any attempt is made to operate the crane.

Mechanical cranes can be fitted with either a bosun's chair or a special carrier that can be used as a stretcher. After the first guard on the scene has gone down on the sky genie to administer urgently needed medical aid, send the next man down in the bosun's chair with additional equipment as needed (i.e., blankets, splints, and resuscitator). Be sure the guard going over the cliff has on necessary safety equipment (gloves, helmet, safety line, three-inch webbing attached to hook). If necessary have the descending guard take down a communicating device (bull horn, walkie-talkie).

When the guard in the chair is no longer in sight, have a guard in an observation position to help direct the descent. This man is usually off to one side where he can observe the entire rescue area. Lower away on command of the man in the chair. At this point the man in the chair is in command; heed his every request.

If a carrier/stretcher is to be used, the procedure is as follows:

1. Carrier must be fitted with a rope adapter (spider web) in order to be lowered down the cliff. After attachment secure to boom hook.
2. Before lowering the carrier, attach guideline and secure all rescue equipment.
3. Once stretcher is down, the victim should be placed in it and securely strapped in position.
4. If a guard is to ride up with the victim, make sure a safety line is worn.

Night Lighting

In order to make an effective cliff rescue in darkness, lighting equipment is a necessity. The following recommended equipment list will cover almost any night cliff rescue operation.

1. One 3000-watt generator;
2. Two electrical tripods with 500-watt bulbs, fifty feet of line (two tripod weight);
3. One copper ground rod;
4. Two yellow waterproof flashlights;
5. One sixty-foot copper ground wire;
6. Two seventy-foot extension cords;

7. One electrical supply box, including One generator jumper cable, Two hand spotlights (twelve volts), One electrical adapter;
8. Two 300-watt lightbulbs (spare);
9. One fog lighting supply box, including Two orange glass filters, Two 500-watt lightbulbs; and
10. One 200-foot portable electrical reel.

Setting up night lighting requires the following procedure:

1. Location of victim will dictate where you set up lighting equipment. Try to extend your tripod lights to form a "T" in order to fully light the area.
2. Once lights are in place, hammer copper ground rod into ground eighteen inches, if possible, to insure a good ground. Hook up ground to generator.
3. Start generator first before plugging lights in. Having the lights plugged in first can produce an overload condition on the generator making it hard to start.
4. Plug lights in and readjust tripods to obtain maximum lighting.
5. When using extension cords, try to use the least amount of footage possible. This will help relieve the load on the generator.
6. If used on a windy night, place tripod weights on the windward side of tripod feet, to prevent tripod from being blown over.
7. If foggy, use orange filters. The orange fog filter will aid in cutting down the glare that's normally reflected back by the fog.
8. Cautions: The generator puts out 115 volts. Always check ground for proper connection. Keep crowds away from lights and cords.

Planning the Cliff Rescue

In order to make a successful cliff operation, plan for the unexpected. Regardless of circumstances, a cliff rescue is a team effort. All parties must be aware of the rescue plan. Points to be included in a rescue plan are outlined below.

1. Condition of victim. The condition of the victim will dictate the rescue plan. Can he walk? Must he be carried? The condition will also dictate if he can survive a leisurely evacuation or if it must be fast.
2. Time of day
   a. Water Glare. When stationing an observation man, take into account, if possible, the glare of the water.
   b. Tidal Flow. If victim is found or rescue is conducted on a reef normally covered during high tide, try to find out the tidal flow. An incoming tide might hinder rescue plans.
3. Weather
   a. Wind effect
      i. Whether a helicopter is to be used or not may depend on wind conditions.
      ii. Dust from the up draft will hinder vision—use goggles.
      iii. When a carrier is being hoisted by boom on a very windy day it may be necessary to use more guide lines for stability.

iv. Updraft and noise created by the wind can hinder communication.

4. Geographical conditions. The geography of the site will be a major factor in evacuation. The use of walking- boom, or M.A. System will be decided upon. The guard must also decide if it is best to ascend or descend with the victim. If there is room, a helicopter might be used and possibly could land. If the site is located near an accessible area by water, a rescue boat could be used.

5. Personnel and Transportation. In planning the rescue, the number of necessary personnel must be determined. Estimates should be liberal, but caution must be taken not to strip guarded beaches.

The rescue plan must be based on, and stress, the following rules:

1. Safety. The rescue plan should be safe for the victim and the rescuers. There will always be an element of risk when working around cliffs.
2. Simplicity. The rescue plan should be the simplest way to do the job. Avoid setting up elaborate lowering or raising systems if there is a simpler way. The less complicated the procedure, the less chance of something going wrong.
3. Swiftness. There is usually plenty of time to evacuate a victim. However, the rescue plan should attempt to remove the victim in the shortest time consistent with safety and simplicity. Some injuries or medical emergencies (cerebral hemorrhage, poisoning, internal injuries, pulmonary edema, appendicitis) require immediate evacuation. The leader must recognize these emergencies.

The following equipment is recommended for a fully operational cliff rescue vehicle:

One resuscitator
Two green splints
One hair traction splint
Three oxygen bottles
Three wood splints (sizes 26″, 34″, and 46″)
One back board splint
One raincoat
Two helmets with two goggles
Two pairs leather gloves
One pair rubber gloves
Two waterproof flashlights
Two blankets
One audiohailer, battery operated
Two faceplates with two snorkels
One tool box with assorted tools
Two pairs tennis shoes
Six flares
One large first aid box
One four-quart canteen
One pack blow-up splints
Two floating chocks
Two round nose shovels

Four round metal stakes
Two flat metal stakes
Two electrical tripods with 500-watt bulbs, fifty-foot line
Two electrical tripod weights
Two sledgehammers
One tow chain
One copper ground rod
One bolt cutter
One crowbar
One sixty-foot copper ground wire
Two seventy-two-foot yellow extension cords
One 150-foot sky genie with two harnesses and packs
One 250-foot sky genie line and pack
One Electrical supply box, including one generator jumper cable, two hand spot light (12-volt), one electrical adapter, one spare battery
One Fog lighting supply box, including two spare lightbulbs, two orange glass filters
Two spare lightbulbs in boxes
One climbing hardware pack, including twelve carabiners (five locking, seven nonlocking), two breaking bars, two pulleys (aluminum), three 9-mm perlon lines, four six-foot, one-inch flat webbing, five ten-foot, one-inch flat nylon webbing
One eighty-four 9-mm polypropane guide line
One 200-foot 10-mm goldline
One 100-foot 10-mm goldline
One seventeen-foot rope ladder
Two 100-foot 9-mm guide lines, plus miscellaneous line, such as 100-foot 12-mm nylon line, eighty-four-foot 9-mm nylon line
One spider web
One bosun's chair
One pair of goggles
One Thompson carrier
One 3000-watt generator
One boat hook
One 200-foot portable electrical reel
Two five pound fire extinguishers, serial
Two 140-foot stake lines
One forty-foot stake line
One twelve-volt hand spot light
One pair 7 x 35 binoculars
One small metal fuse box with assorted fuses.

6

COMMUNICATIONS AND BACKUP SYSTEMS

GENERAL PHILOSOPHY

The most vital auxiliary function performed by any marine safety or lifeguard service is communications. A well-organized and efficiently run centralized communications system is an absolute necessity in a large organization that services a vast geographical location and employs a complex backup system. Even the smallest type of lifeguard operation can and should utilize a few of the basic procedures.

The primary functions of communications are threefold.

1. To provide lifeguard personnel, whether they be in towers, mobile vehicles, or vessels or on foot patrol, with the ability to communicate with each other in an expedient and efficient manner;
2. To provide operational supervision with the ability to coordinate all emergency activities within the scope of the service and with mutual agencies such as the local Coast Guard, police, and fire departments and other lifeguard services; and
3. To enforce beach rules and regulations and aid the public by advising them of the hazards of potentially dangerous locations and situations.

An effective communications system is the result of teamwork, necessitating each individual's utmost concentration, alertness, and complete understanding of operational procedures. The key forms of communication are intercommunicable telephone and radio systems, public address facilities, hand and whistle signals, and flag systems.

TELEPHONE SYSTEMS

The use of some type of telephone system is a must for any service that employs two or more personnel covering a relatively vast area in which they are out of voice range. Larger organizations should utilize a centralized PBX (private branch exchange) switchboard linking all towers on an intercommunicable basis. This system is a little more expensive, but has several desirable advantages, especially for a large-scale beach operation. Each station can be contacted individually or as part of a group. In addition, direct lines can be established with the Coast Guard, police, and other mutual agencies. Modern push-button phone systems are available that eliminate the switchboard operator. While this type of system may work well for a relatively small operation, it is not generally advisable for moderate to large service, since it bypasses headquarters' personnel and severely hampers their ability to coordinate and supervise major emergencies. Due to the corrosive elements of the salt air indigenous to ocean beaches, it is strongly advised that said systems be installed underground.

Suggested General Rules

1. Conversations should be brief and accurate, and code should be used whenever possible.
2. Phones should not be used by the public except in cases of emergency.
3. Personal calls of a nonemergency nature should be strongly discouraged.
4. When answering the telephone, guards should give their tower number and last name.
5. Switchboard operators in particular should cultivate a courteous tone and be sure the requested information is given. Calls that they are unable to answer or calls from news media should be referred to a supervisor.

Suggested Tower Procedure

1. When requesting to speak to another tower, the lifeguard picks up the phone, and when the dispatcher answers, gives him the number or name of the tower he wishes to speak with. When that tower answers, the guard will give him his tower number or name and then his last name.

2. When leaving on a rescue or other emergency, the lifeguard knocks the receiver from the phone and taps three times on the phone button or hook.
3. When he needs to request specific emergency equipment, he taps the phone button or hook six times. The dispatcher will drop all calls to answer. (This method should be used in only extreme emergencies, such as resuscitation cases, mass rescues, gang fights, and riots.)
4. When a lifeguard needs assistance and has time to ask for it, he gives the dispatcher all the necessary information relative to the nature and location as time will allow.

RADIO SYSTEMS

Radio systems for intercommunication between mobile units and a central communication center are also necessary equipment in any public safety organization. While any size service would be better off in most instances with their own frequencies, smaller services, due to economics, will most often be a part of a city or county police or fire radio network. Large-scale operations should make every effort to have their own frequencies, as well as separate auxiliary channels that provide contact with other mutual agencies such as the Coast Guard and local fire and police agencies. Irregardless of the type of system utilized, it is imperative to comply with established regulations since most radio communications are monitored by federal agencies.

Lifeguard vehicles and vessels should be assigned to functions and areas that relate to geographic divisions. If there are two or more agencies operating on one frequency, it is strongly recommended that a two-channel operation be incorporated. One channel could then be utilized strictly for emergency traffic and formal dispatching and the other for nonemergency and administrative communications.

FCC Regulations

Many countries have established regulations that govern licensed two-way radio use. In the United States, the regulatory agency is the Federal Communications Commission (FCC), which has rules that must be strictly obeyed. A violation may result in severe penalties to the person(s) responsible.

1. The operator of a base station may turn the set off and on, but must not make any adjustments or repairs. Under no circumstances is the set to be opened.
2. No person shall damage or permit to be damaged any radio equipment in a licensed radio station.

3. No person shall transmit any unnecessary, unidentified, or super-fluous radio communications or signals. Only the assigned call letters and unit numbers shall be used.
4. No person shall transmit any false call letters or any false signals or messages.
5. No person shall transmit communications containing any obscene or profane words, language, or meaning.
6. No person shall interfere with or cause interference with any radio communication or signal.
7. No person shall obtain, attempt to obtain, or help another to obtain an operator's license by fraudulent means.
8. The operator of every base station shall give the assigned call letters at the end of each call.
9. The operator of a mobile unit shall give his unit number at the beginning of each call.
10. Every operator shall obey all the lawful orders concerning the use of the radio network.

Rules For General Operation

1. Pronounce words distinctly and slowly.
2. Control the voice to show as little emotion as possible on the air, regardless of the situation. Emotion tends to distort the voice. Attempt to make the voice a monotone. No experience is required, only a high degree of intelligible and factual information.
3. Keep mouth close to the microphone and speak in a natural tone. Do not shout. The radio itself provides the necessary amplification.
4. Be impersonal on the air and refrain from using the name of the person spoken to. Operators should not refer to themselves as "I".
5. Do not guess! Check all doubtful words with sender. Never transmit 10-4 (OK or acknowledgement) for a message until definitely certain of all details.
6. Give all numbers as an individual number and then repeated in sequence.
7. When dispatching a unit to an emergency, designate a definite response code (i.e., Code One, Two, or Three).
8. Maintain radio logs listing every call transmitted and/or received. Responsibility for this function lies directly with the communication officer.

Tips On Mobile Operation

1. When making a radio call, do not park under a metal roof shed or inside a steel building. In the fringe areas, do not park underneath trees, immediately adjacent to steel structures, or underneath dense overhead wiring.
2. If having trouble being heard, rev up the engine while transmitting.
3. On vehicles provided with a combination electronic siren and a public address system, the guard must make sure to use the radio microphone and not the public address microphone.

4. If the red "transmit" light remains on when not transmitting, this is an indication of equipment trouble. The guard must check to see that the mike button is not stuck. If this is not the trouble, the guard should immediately turn the radio off and report the trouble to the base station.

Emergency Procedure

If possible, always call a base station for emergency messages and relate as much of the following information as possible.

1. The nature of the emergency,
2. The exact location, and
3. What equipment and/or personnel are needed.

In all cases of emergency, the guard must be sure to get all the information he can obtain. The lifeguard must be sure that the receiving operator has received the message correctly. He must stay near the radio set, if possible, to give additional information if required.

Base Station Log

The station log is a permanent record that should contain specific information about each transmission in which the base station participates. The daily log sheet is divided into columns with specific headings and should be completely filled for each call. This sheet is normally retained for a period of seven years or more, primarily for legal purposes. Column headings are:

1. Date (month and day of call),
2. Time (hour and minute of call),
3. Unit contacted,
4. Nature of call (brief resumen of call), and
5. Time call was completed.

In order to conserve air time and yet insure accurate and concise transmissions, specific code terms should be used.

PUBLIC ADDRESS SYSTEMS

Public address systems are widely used at the great majority of beaches. They are an excellent tool for control of the public through means of general announcements and directions. The use of PA systems should be limited to important and necessary information and directions. Most announcements should be repeated two or three times to prevent possible misunderstanding. Training in the proper use of the microphone and the voice is important. These systems must be powerful enough to overcome adverse winds and other obstructions. In selecting a PA system for a salt water environment, corrosive tolerance is a prime factor.

Speaker-siren units for beach mobile units and vessels have also proved to be very efficient communication tools. Several such systems are available, many effective up to a quarter mile or more. In addition to providing public address capability, these systems are equipped with electronic sirens. Also, when a guard has to respond to a location several yards away from his unit, he can switch his radio to the outside speaker.

Self-contained portable address systems of the small hand-held variety are a handy tool for the individual lifeguard working a small semiremote or remote area. Most are effective up to about 200 yards. However, their use on beaches is limited due to their range capacity.

FLAG, SIGN, AND HAND COMMUNICATIONS

Whistle and hand signals are a vital means of communication at any beach. The shrill police type whistle is generally needed to call attention to the lifeguard. It is important to use the whistle sparingly and only when needed. When communicating with other guards, it is of utmost importance that a definite whistle code be established so that there can be no mistakes in your message. A common procedure is to use only one long whistle for a "stand by" and three short whistles indicating a need for immediate response. Once contact is made, both parties can communicate with hand signals.

On the following pages appear examples of the standard flag, sign and hand communications.

BACKUP SYSTEM

It is of vital importance that a backup system be established at any beach regardless of the number of lifeguards on duty. When a lifeguard leaves his post or station to make a rescue, tend a first aid, or for any other reason, the area he is responsible for must be watched by another lifeguard. This cannot be left to chance or haphazard arrangement. A system must be devised whereby each area is guarded, and none is left unguarded. One bathing accident will very often tend to panic others in the vicinity, leading to the possibility of one or more additional incidents. The exact way in

SWIMMING PERMITTED
Black figure on white background with green circle.

SWIMMING PROHIBITED
Black figure on white background with red circle and diagonal.

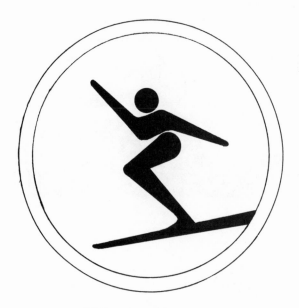

SURFING PERMITTED
Black figure on white background with green circle.

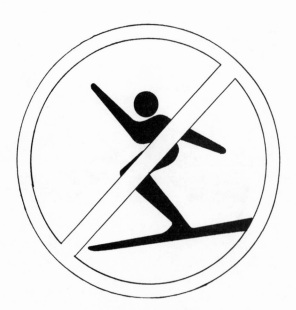

SURFING PROHIBITED
Black figure on white background with red circle and diagonal.

SIGNALS FROM WATER

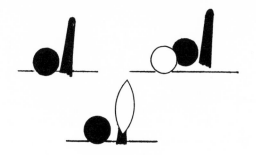

HELP OR ASSISTANCE REQUIRED
(By swimmer, beltman, boardman, etc.)
Raise, hold and lower after a few seconds.

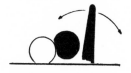

RESUSCITATION REQUIRED
Arm—single wave at intervals

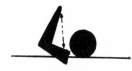

PAY OUT LINE
Flexing motion of arm—3 times.

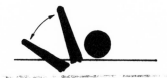

HAUL IN LINE
Raised arm brought downward—beating the water—3 times.

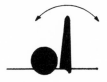

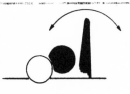

STOP
Double wave at intervals until stop results.

DISGARDED SAFETY BELT
Treble wave at intervals until *understood*. If mistaken for stop, the results will not be serious.

SIGNALS FROM SHORE

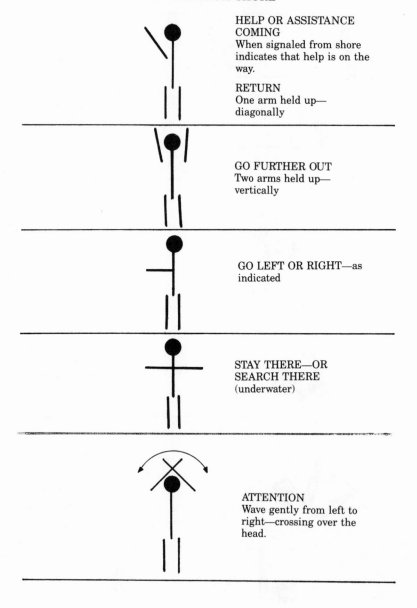

HELP OR ASSISTANCE
COMING
When signaled from shore
indicates that help is on the
way.

RETURN
One arm held up—
diagonally

GO FURTHER OUT
Two arms held up—
vertically

GO LEFT OR RIGHT—as
indicated

STAY THERE—OR
SEARCH THERE
(underwater)

ATTENTION
Wave gently from left to
right—crossing over the
head.

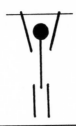

WAIT OUTSIDE SURF
Pole, oar, towel or other
object held between the
raised arms.

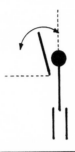

SHARK (where needed)
or
RETURN—EMERGENCY
(where no sharks)
Wave furiously from water,
shore or craft.

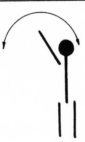

ALL CLEAR (from shore,
water, boat, or other craft)
Wave slowly in half circle to
right.

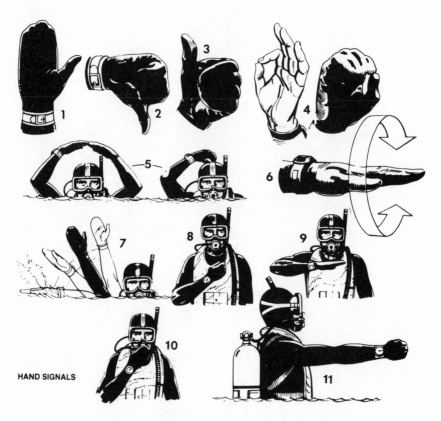

HAND SIGNALS

SKIN AND SCUBA DIVING HAND SIGNALS

NO.	SIGNAL	MEANING	COMMENT
1.	Hand raised, fingers pointed up, palm to receiver	Stop	Transmitted the same as a traffic policeman's STOP
2.	Thumb extended downward from clenched fist	Go down or Going down	

3. Thumb extended upward from clenched fist	Go up or Going up	
4. Thumb and forefinger making a circle with 3 remaining fingers extended if possible	OK! or OK?	Divers wearing mittens may not be able to distinctly extend 3 remaining fingers (see both drawings of signal)
5. Two arms extended overhead with fingertips touching above head to make a large O shape	OK! or OK?	A diver with only one arm free may make this signal by extending that arm overhead with fingertips touching top of head to make the O shape. Signal is for long range
6. Hand flat, fingers together, palm down, thumb sticking out, then hand rocking back and forth on axis of forearm	Something is wrong	This is the opposite of OK! The signal does not indicate an emergency
7. Hand waving overhead (may also thrash hand on water)	Distress	Indicates immediate aid required
8. Fist pounding on chest	Low on air	Indicates signaler's air supply is reduced to the quantity agreed upon in predive planning
9. Hand slashing or chopping throat	Out of air	Indicates that signaler cannot breathe for some reason
10. Fingers pointing to mouth	Let's Buddy Breathe	The regulator may be either in or out of the mouth
11. Clenched fist on arm extended in direction of danger	Danger	

Shore Flags

All flags to be not less than 30 inches by 24 inches in size, except where otherwise indicated, and flown on flagpoles so sited and in such numbers that they are readily seen by any person in or approaching the swimming area.

SHARK

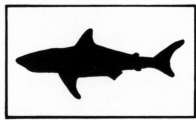

White background with black figure

RED FLAG

Whenever swimming is considered to be temporarily unsafe, this should be so indicated by flying the *red flag*.

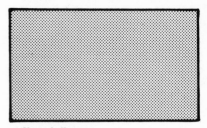

All red flag

PATROLLED AREA

Areas under close and continuous supervision and surveillance by lifeguards. The *red and yellow flags* should be flown in pairs (or greater numbers) to indicate the patrolled area.

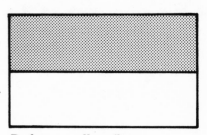

Red over yellow flag

DIVING FLAG

Diver below or in the immediate area. Usually flown on a float (with a staff of not less than 3 feet) over the area in which divers are below the surface.

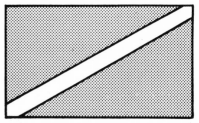

White diagonal stripe across a red flag

BLACK BALL FLAG

During times when the *black ball flag* is flown, swimming only is permitted in an area adjacent to the beach within 200 yards of the point of display. When the *black ball flag* is displayed from consecutive operational lifeguard towers, stations, or similar structures, all waters adjacent to the beach in that area are restricted to swimming and bathing only.

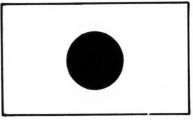

Yellow rectangular flag with a solid black circle in the center, 1 foot in diameter

SIGNAL FLAGS

These flags are to be used in pairs. The colors should be bright yellow and flourescent red. The flags are to be used for signals only and give no meaning to the general public. *Size: 18 inches by 24 inches.*

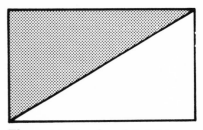

Flourescent red and bright yellow diagonals

which any backup system is set up will depend on the location and distances between guarding towers, the number of personnel available, and the type of mobile equipment utilized.

A backup system goes in effect every time a guard leaves his tower or may go into effect on a signal from a tower or, in a highly advanced operation, via the telephone and/or radio. The guarding of a large ocean beach area will necessitate a highly advanced and complex backup system. The extent will be dependent on a number of factors—visitation, geographical environment, prevailing weather and surf conditions, and the nature of the water recreational activities.

Mobile Vehicle Support

The use of mobile units on most beach areas of any comparable size are a must. A four-wheel drive mobile unit can respond quickly to the great majority of water or beach emergencies. Other advantages are storage of rescue and first aid supplies and equipment not to mention transportation of additional manpower.

Mobile Vessel Support

Large, heavily populated beach areas, especially those subject to heavy surf and riptide activity, should strongly consider the use of high speed rescue vessels as supplementary backup support. These vessels can maintain maximum response times regardless of dense beach population, which can severely hamper the response capabilities of mobile beach vehicles. Rescue vessels have also proved to be a most effective means of rescuing swimmers outside the surfline and for protecting swimmers and other persons from pleasure craft that drift into the surfline because of either mechanical problems or operator negligence. In areas where high cliffs prevail and there is little beach area, the use of some type of vessel may be the only feasible method of patrol.

Central Tower Support

An extremely popular method for providing observational backup is the central guarding tower. Many beaches employ main towers at a location that provides a broad viewing scope of the entire geographic area. Where possible, a pier, jetty, or natural point can be used. From such a vantage point, one man can visually protect several miles of beach, and when emergencies arise, he is in a position to view them and direct mobile backup units or additional flanking tower guards to the scene. This particular central vantage tower is equipped with a high-powered telescope, public address system, and radio and telephone communications.

RECOMMENDED BACKUP PROCEDURE

1. Beach unit operation with fully staffed towers
   a. A preventative effort is preferred to avoid total commitment.
   b. Surveillance is maintained when tower guards are committed.
   c. Additional support is provided to tower guards on multiple victim rescues.
   d. One man remains with the unit until the last moment to retain visual coverage of the area.
   e. The unit will make a rescue if it is directly on scene between two towers and immediate response is vital.
2. Beach unit operation with partial tower staffing
   a. The unit assumes a greater role as a mobile tower in addition to a support function.
   b. The unit operator must position the unit where response is likely to be needed and constantly reassess the position in relation to shifting areas of probable activity.
   c. Stationing the vehicle at towers in operation or with other units is avoided.
   d. Unit remains in the high activity area and does not patrol the activity area unnecessarily.
   e. If rescue vessels are in service, beach units should avoid duplicate coverage.
3. Beach unit operation with no towers
   a. Any movement of the unit other than shifting attention or responding to preventative actions should be avoided, since water-oriented emphasis is greatly impaired when patrolling.
   b. Closed towers should be utilized as a base for spotting when conditions permit, to enhance visual efficiency when possible.
4. Land and sea units, coordinated rescue (no towers staffed)
   a. Guards should keep in mind that when both a vessel and a beach unit guard are committed, the beach is guarded solely by the boat operator. As a result, speed is of utmost importance in executing the rescue.
   b. Land unit—primary response. The vessel crew must monitor the situation to determine if a backup is needed. If the vessel is not busy, the victim should be taken to it to relieve the land unit guard and facilitate his rapid return to the beach.
   c. Sea unit—primary response. The land unit must monitor the situation to determine if a backup is needed. In cases of multiple victims close to the neck of the riptide, a land unit response is almost always necessary. It is the land unit's responsibility to be in close proximity to respond quickly if needed.
   d. Land and sea units—coordinated rescue response. The land unit generally has the major responsibility for rescue inside the surfline. The sea unit is generally more effective in the area outside the surfline.

The following diagram illustrates the potential of the land, sea, and control tower perimeter defense and mobile backup system when utilized to its fullest degree. While a central tower located on a pier can provide much greater observational capability because of elevation and angle factors, in the absence of a pier, the control tower could be placed near any centralized location offering the most advantageous height and angle. Advantages of utilizing ocean rescue vessels for mobile backup are shown in the diagram. Note how quickly the rescue vessel could respond to the emergency area if additional manpower were needed. The rescue vessel would be in a position to dispatch additional personnel in much less time than other procedures would normally take. It should be remembered that although the guards aboard the vessel could be utilized, it will not be necessary to have flanking towers respond and further deplete beachfront coverage. The guard in the central tower has high-powered telescopes and a public address system and is in the best position to supervise the rescue operation, directing guards and comforting victims with the PA system, if necessary. If the rescue involves an inshore hole or small rip, the responsibility for primary backup would then shift to the land unit.

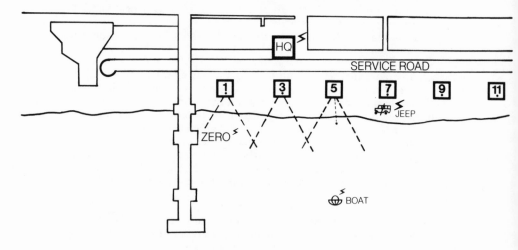

7

Underwater Search and Recovery

Lack of oxygen is the cause of death by drowning and also can cause brain damage in some revived victims. Brain damage may vary in severity from a temporary state to a permanent condition and is caused by deterioration of the brain cells. Deterioration can take place when the body has been deprived of air for only about four minutes, depending on the age and physical condition of the victim. Records show that persons submerged for as long as a half hour have survived with little or no brain damage.

Most drownings take place near shore, usually just out of safety's reach. In the still waters of bays and ponds, drownings most often occur where sudden changes of depth cause the nonswimmer to lose touch with the bottom and panic. At surf beaches, the greatest percentage of drownings result from persons exhausting themselves fighting currents and waves. When a person panics in the water, it is said that he has one foot in the doorway of death. It is a fact that panic, including the loss of ability to act or make judgments, is the greatest cause of all drownings.

There are two basic types of drowning situations. One is the skilled person who finds himself in water he can't handle. He is capable of waving, shouting, or showing signs of distress that attract watchers on the beach. The other is the nonswimmer who suddenly can't touch bottom. He cannot wave because he lacks the swimming skill to support himself, and he cannot shout because he is frantically gasping for breath. The trained guard can quickly spot (1) a victim facing the beach or nearest object that might support him; (2) arm movements that thrash the water, usually with both arms extended laterally.

These arm movements cannot propel the victim in any direction, but merely raise and lower him in the water as he tries to gulp air. As the drowning progresses, the victim's head sinks lower and lower in the water. His arms become less visible and their movement more feeble until only the top of his head and grasping hands can be seen. Sometimes as a last resort, a physically strong nonswimmer will try to float on his back. Thus, the total drowning process can be lengthy or immediate.

Buoyancy varies with individual physical build—for example, light or heavy bone structure and a fat body versus a muscular one. A person with excess fat tends to be quite buoyant. Clothing is another factor to consider. A clothed person will be dragged underwater as the fabric absorbs moisture; in contrast, with wet suits, increasing thickness of the material allows increased buoyancy. Thus, not all drowned or near-drowned persons are found on the bottom; they may be suspended in midwater or even float on the surface. Water having an extraordinarily high salt content is likely to buoy a floating body to a point at or near the surface.

Because of these variables, some persons struggle on the surface before slipping underwater, while others sink almost at once. Very few call out for help; they enter death silently when panic deprives them of their reason.

HYPERVENTILATION

A guard going to the rescue of a victim who has disappeared underwater, swims his head high and eyes fixed on the last spot at which he saw the victim. This procedure is, of course, followed in any rescue but is crucial in drowning. The guard must hyperventilate as he approaches the area where the victim was last seen. Hyperventilation—that is, excessive breathing in and out to reduce the carbon dioxide in the system—prepares the body for the dive by enabling one to stay underwater for periods longer than normally possible. This technique is dangerous if repeated overlong as it can cause a chemical imbalance within the body, resulting in unpredictable unconsciousness. The correct way to hyperventilate is to stay calm strive for relaxation, breathe out more air than is breathed in, and repeat taking three to five deep breaths and exhalations before submerging. The guard must keep a clear head while searching for the victim by fighting excitement and surface at once if he begins to feel more comfortable than he should after a considerable period of submerging.

LANDMARKS

If the victim cannot be located at once, at least two sets of landmarks on the shore should be selected to fix the location. One set fixes the line perpendicular to the beach and the other the distance from the waterline at the spot where the victim was last seen. With this fix, the guard cannot lose the prime search area as he is moved by the current, waves, or misjudgment. After selecting the landmarks, the guard makes a series of short dives, about fifteen to twenty seconds each, sweeping the immediate area. Between dives, he checks the landmarks to prevent wandering from the sight. In diving, the hands must be stretched out before the diver when visibility is limited—and especially any time that a faceplate is not worn. If the water is deeper than the length of the rescue buoy line (about six feet), the guard should unsnap the line and discard the unit.

BRINGING THE VICTIM TO THE SURFACE

There is no single recommended method for bringing a victim to the surface, except that the head first seems natural and may be easier because the limbs fall into a streamlined position.

USE OF AIRCRAFT

Bodies are difficult to locate, especially in dirty water and areas of current or wave action. Any aircraft, but particularly a helicopter, is a tremendous asset in the search. Its high vantage point over the water offers a wide scope of visibility, and often the crew can see slight changes in bottom shadings that indicate the presence of a victim. A description of the victim's clothing is most helpful to the flying search team, as the whole body is seldom seen at once, but a bit of color can lead to recognition of its location.

SEARCH TEAM WORK

When more than one lifeguard is available for an underwater search, teamwork is crucial and effective. The more personnel, the greater the area that can be covered in the shortest possible time. All the guards work as a unit with one leader designated. When a victim has first gone under, one guard and his backup generally initiate the rescue. As the search continues, backup support personnel arrive, and diving equipment is brought in. An organized search team enters the water, and one man remains on the beach in charge of radio and public address communications. The leader's task is (1) calling for additional personnel or gear; (2) guiding aircraft or boat search personnel; (3) providing arriving personnel with the accident details, location of the victim, best water entry and exit points, description of the victim's clothes, the rescue search plan, who is in charge; (4) keeping bathers and swimmers out of the area; (5) guarding the equipment on the beach against theft; and (6) issuing "disregard" advice to personnel en route if the victim is found.

CARE OF VICTIM'S LOVED ONES

Relatives, friends, or loved ones of the victim should be watched and cared for. They may be in a state of severe traumatic shock or try to participate in the search, only to become victims of drowning or near-drowning themselves.

LENGTH OF SEARCHES

The search should continue until a ranking officer decides that it is fruitless—usually an hour after the known starting time. The precise time that the search began must be noted accurately, never estimated; excitement can cause miscalculation. The only part of the search that is discontinued is the diving operation. Aircraft and boats that have been called to assist may continue until dark.

During the entire rescue operation, lifeguard observation posts must remain manned. Too often, concentration on the search by all guards in or near the area causes duplication of effort or neglect of other important duties. All water recreation in the search area is stopped to prevent confusion.

Many drownings occur away from guarded areas, but within the jurisdiction of a lifeguard agency. The time and personnel alloted for such searches depend upon the conditions at the guarded beaches and the manpower available, at the discretion of the designated lifeguard in charge.

USE OF A RESCUE VESSEL

Lifeguard rescue boats may play a role in search endeavors, but their capability is limited in the surf zone. They can, however, locate rip current heads visually by scanning the surface. They can provide additional personnel and equipment at or near the drowning site and provide support for crowd control and rescue communications by means of their public address system.

Rescue boats are often utilized in the search and recovery procedures when a rough surf is not involved. By towing divers holding on to a twenty-foot pole in a horizontal altitude to the transom, and just off the ocean floor, very large areas may be covered in a short period of time. This method does not fatigue the diver. Divers are assigned in accordance with visibility. In other words, if the visibility is five feet, only four divers are necessary to cover the twenty-foot span of the pole. The boat operator must always remember that he is in charge of maintaining strict search patterns as well as suitable speeds, usually under three knots.

INLAND WATER SEARCHES

Lifeguard agencies are often asked by local law enforcement officials to search inland waters, such as lakes, ponds, or reservoirs, that are within their jurisdiction and are thought to contain a body or object related to a crime. This is dangerous work. Visibility is limited or nonexistent. Trash, brush, or barbed wire on the bottom can easily snag a diver; and he may be caught or seriously injured and drown.

The composition of lakes and ponds varies widely, and the bottom may have spongy mud overgrown with grass and moss. Many have sunken logs, cars, tires, bed springs, or other debris. Attempting to conduct a thorough search while navigating around hazardous obstacles is a dangerous task even with scuba gear. The growth can snare a harness or leg, completely immobilizing an unwary diver.

In manmade ponds or lakes, the bottom composition is mud, sometimes many feet thick. Reservoirs are notable for the thickness of the mud bottom. The object of a search may be partially buried. A respectable distance must be maintained from all pipe outlets because their strong suction can actually entrap a diver. With scuba gear, a diver should remain attached to a safety line to the surface; however, the safest rule is complete avoidance of all pipes.

All inland waters that contain fish also contain the implements of fishing. The most dangerous items are lures and hooks attached to lengths of monofilament line. The line is very difficult to see, and if entangled, the diver may need assistance from a buddy to free himself. Waters surrounding piers, docks, and anchorages most often contain these items. Never drag yourself along the bottom or rake your bare hands through the bottom, as broken glass and other sharp articles can inflict wounds. In bays, near shore waters, and in other water channels, stingrays lie resting on the bottom almost completely covered by sand or mud.

Rivers contain all the aforementioned dangers except stingrays and in addition have strong currents. Extreme caution and thoughtful search planning are essential in these waterways. Rivers vary so widely in size, width, depth, current velocity, and bottom topography that no two search efforts are ever identical. It is recommended that recovery work be avoided during storm and flood conditions, waiting until the swelling water recedes.

Bays, too, are obstacle laden and have swift currents during tidal changes; however, the visibility is clearest when the incoming tide brings fresh sea water to dilute silt-filled bay water. Visibility decreases during the tidal ebb. Back bays usually stay dirty, since they lack fresh sea water circulation and are subject to increased plankton bloom.

Bay bottoms are muddiest nearest the shore and increasingly sandy closest to the ocean entrance. Swimming coves remain dirty when in use because sediment is constantly kicked up from the floor by bathers. When searching the bottom of any waterway, disturb the bottom as little as possible. Sand or mud remains suspended in the water for considerable time and decreases the visibility.

To dive in dirty but nonsurf areas, after an initial few dives to determine the visibility and best procedure, gloves should be worn to protect the guard's hands from sharp objects. (Where surf exists, most sharp objects have been rubbed smooth by sand and small rocks, with the exception of newly deposited refuse.)

USE OF GRAPNEL IRONS

If visibility is exceptionally poor, the diving search may have to be abandoned in favor of a bottom search by means of a boat and grapnel iron. The proper type of iron is selected for the job, and it is dropped to the bottom and slowly dragged in a decided pattern over the search area. When the grapnel operator feels a pull, indicating that some object has been snagged, the boat is stopped, and the object is raised and examined. Sometimes it is necessary to send a diver down to investigate the object by feel, if it cannot be raised, or to unsnag the grapnel if it is merely entangled. Trash that is brought to the surface should be removed from the search area, as it will undoubtedly be snagged repeatedly, slowing the search operation.

The grapnels most often used are (1) the gang grapnel, a series of large, triple, nonbarbed hooks spaced on a bar or pipe not less than three feet in length that is pulled behind and parallel to the transom of the boat; and (2) the single grapnel, an anchor with more than three pointed flukes weighing about fifteen to twenty pounds. Both grapnels should be attached to a length of chain to ensure that they drag on the bottom. The gang grapnel is best for retrieving bodies, and the single grapnel is excellent for handling solid objects. The grapnel method is useless on rocky terrain or in areas of heavy kelp or sea grass growth.

USE OF SCUBA GEAR

Self-contained underwater breathing apparatus can be of great value in prolonged underwater searches, deep water work, inspections, recovery operations, and related ventures. In emergencies when time is of the essence, however, its weight and bulk and/or the length of time needed to rig could prove to be detrimental factors. Most drownings take place in less than twenty feet of water, and a skin diver can cover as much ground as a tank diver. Sometimes the free diver is more effective because he is more agile without the weight of scuba gear; he can work safely in white water where a tank diver cannot; and in clear water he can conduct his search from the surface, where use of a mask and snorkel permits him a wide overview of the terrain. In a prolonged search, where there is limited visibility but little surf, a team of scuba divers can be more effective, especially if the water depth is more than twenty feet. As in all rescues or recoveries, a full description of the body or object—particularly its color—is of primary value.

NIGHT WATER SEARCHES

Underwater searches at night should be restricted to cases of extreme emergency. After a well-organized attempt, the search should be discontinued until the following morning. Floodlighting at the surface or from a boat's bridge is a tremendous asset. It helps the surface team or supervisor to see how effective the underwater search pattern is and aids underwater visibility. Underwater flashlights used by the swimming guards should have sealed beam construction and not be so buoyant as to hinder the underwater worker. These lights should be checked after every dive for leakage and battery power; obviously, weak light diminishes their usefulness.

OCEAN SEARCHES

In our variable oceans, the main problems in a search are surf and currents. Visibility changes radically from area to area and day to day. Rip currents, which are responsible for so many drownings, are filled with suspended sediment stirred up by the water movement and lack visibility. In some areas of heavy surf, there is never a clearance of white water. Here, a body may periodically boil to the surface, only to disappear once again. Surface scanning, in this instance, is as important as diving, and often the underwater search may be by feel.

In preparation for an underwater search, a full description of the body or object to be located and where it was last seen are needed. Colors, shape, and weight are crucial elements of description. The first guard at the accident scene may have to depend on eyewitnesses for information. Since they are excited and often unreliable, the guard's experienced interpretation of the information is essential. In the event of no witnesses—for example, a lost child report near a beach area—an educated guess may be effective.

Water clarity, surf, and surge conditions and currents should be closely observed. Most important—choose a safe access. The best entry point into the water is sometimes not the safest exit point back to the beach. In this case, two access points should be chosen and all personnel involved should be told of these locations by the person in charge.

DIVE TEAM TRAINING

Using scuba gear in underwater searches takes coordination and lengthy training. A professional lifeguard service may have a trained scuba squad or may require all of its full-time personnel to be trained to meet special problems in their area of jurisdiction.

Vertigo

The same sensation that gives a diver the feeling of weightlessness in dark water also gives him difficulty in deciphering direction. An untrained diver may not be able to tell which way is up, down, north, or south. Nothing could be worse for search and recovery work, where maintenance of bearing is a necessity. Recommended training to improve this sense is use of blacked out face plates (cover the inside of the glass with foil) in swimming pool exercises. The exercise pattern is swum first with unobstructed masks and then without visibility.

Kick

A diver's kick is hardly ever true. In other words, he kicks harder with one leg than the other. If this is not known and compensated for, swimming will assume a pattern of large, erratic circles when visibility is lacking. Some divers spin like tops when descending toward an unseen bottom. Again, this signifies an uneven kick.

Cold Water

An extreme temperature drop (from air to water) can result in numbness, lack of coordination, and loss of alertness. It drains a swimmer's strength and causes a scuba diver to consume more air. Well-fitted neoprene wetsuits of a thickness to suit the local water temperature are advisable for the dive team. The suits should be dried thoroughly between uses, and if not nylon lined, they should be dusted with powder ready for the next wearing. (Suitable powders are baby powder, talcum powder, or corn starch.) The neoprene suits should never be left in direct sunlight for long periods of time and should be checked periodically for wear and rot.

Weight Belts

Each member of the diving team will learn how much lead weight he needs on a belt, according to expected dive depth and equipment carried, to counteract the buoyancy of his wetsuit.

Tanks (aqualungs)

Thorough training is required for the use and care of scuba equipment. Because it is so easy and pleasant to use, a diver may forget small hazards that can accompany a dive. Scuba tanks should be refilled with air as soon as possible after diving to prevent interior rusting and must be hydrotested and ICC (Interstate Commerce Commission) recertified every three to five years. Brightly colored tanks are an asset underwater in team efforts. Colored wetsuit hoods offer the same safety factor in aiding underwater detection of search team members.

Diving Diseases

As part of their scuba training, the team will learn the symptoms of, signs of, and treatment for all diving diseases. They will become aware of their individual capabilities according to depth. The lifeguard agency should set an absolute depth limit past which their men will not be sent. It is recommended that there be a one hundred-foot depth limit for lifeguard agency dive teams. Depth gauges worn by the guards will keep them informed of their depth from the surface.

Quick Releases

All heavy gear worn by the dive team should have quick release fastenings. This particularly applies to the scuba harness and shoulder straps and the weight belt buckle.

Diving Equipment Locker

All lifeguard agencies should have a diving gear locker in which
to store major equipment. Basic dive gear—fins, masks, snorkels,
gloves, search line (average length about thirty feet), and a small
buoy with a weight—can be kept in mobile units and rescue
vehicles.

The diving gear locker should hold spare basic equipment, plus
scuba tanks, regulators, wetsuits, diving knives, diving compasses,
decompression meters, depth gauges, suit powder, suit repair kits,
weight belts, decompression tables, recharge units for filling scuba
tanks, range poles, grapnel irons, and tools for repair. A melting pot
for heating scrap lead to mold weight belt units is useful.

Specified vehicles may be designated for carrying scuba gear
(tanks and regulators). A rescue boat equipped with complete scuba
gear may be of more value, as it can place a diver beyond the surf
line fully equipped very quickly.

SEARCH LINES

A search line is a multipurpose piece of rope, one-quarter to three-
eighths inches in diameter and brightly colored. Its prime use is to
space out the members of a dive team at a distance where each man
can barely see the man on either side of him. The line is then swum
before them, parallel to their shoulders. This keeps the team
together and spread out on a single line. It is up to each man to see
that his part of the line remains taut. One man, usually the furthest
to the right, is in charge, and signals are passed by a series of
prearranged yanks on the line designating the next maneuver. If the
team is made up of scuba divers, the search pattern can be
controlled either by a preset compass course or by having two
surface swimmers mark the ends of the search line, giving signals to
those below by rope yanks. When search lines are not available, any
cloth or rope can be used to simulate one, but never dive holding
hands. The hands are needed to protect the face and body.

SEARCH EQUIPMENT

Search and recovery divers need simple and practical equipment
that can be utilized in a variety of ways. Signals should be simple,
not complex; they should be reviewed before each dive job. Suggested
signals for rope jerking sequences should indicate (1) speed up, (2)
slow down, (3) stop, (4) surface, and (5) object found.

When searching by compass course, the team will surface before
each course change. Since a well-practiced team can judge distance

by time, an underwater watch will aid the precision of this maneuver.

A free dive team can stay in a given search area more easily than a scuba team, but will be limited by depth and burdened by long and short breath holders. That is, they will surface at different times and places, according to breath-holding capacity. Since those who can hold their breath the longest can travel the furthest underwater, the guard in charge will have to almost reorganize his team after each dive. He will probably have to backtrack each time to the surfacing point of the weakest diver. Breath-holding capacity improves with practice, so planned exercise will benefit the entire crew.

Range Poles

Range poles mark a bearing point of a shore-based search that is dependent upon orientation and control from a focal point. They create one set of landmarks that are obvious to all search members and can be moved according to the progress of the search. Each range pole has a diamond-shaped board mounted at the top of an eight- or ten-foot pole. The face is painted with two contrasting colors. Range poles are used in pairs, so the color pattern used on one pole should be reversed on the other, as demonstrated in the accompanying drawing. They must be large enough to be seen by a surface swimmer at a distance of 300 yards.

It is best to have a search line which is the same length as the sweep being made by the team. This allows the shore-based leaders to measure out the distance for the placement of the next pole placement before the team reaches the end of the first sweep. Then no delay occurs in relocation, and the team need not tread water to wait for a change in bearings.

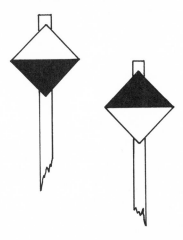

Marker Buoys

Marker buoys are used for a variety of reasons—(1) to outline a search area, (2) to mark the spot where the object of the search was last seen, (3) to mark areas previously searched, (4) to mark water hazards to divers, and (5) to provide markers for boats moving in the area to avoid divers in the water.

When scuba divers are using buoys as a central bearing point, as in a circle search, they should never surface after completion of a sweep without first returning to the anchor buoy rope and following it to the surface. This precludes being run over by a boat, if any are in the area.

Marker buoys should have anchor weights sufficient to hold them in place, but not so heavy as to restrict their movement by a diver. The anchor line should not be too long for the depths in which its use is expected to take place, nor should it have any tails that can tangle in the diver's gear. The anchor line lengths should be set at the site of rescue or recovery operations. Suggested underwater hand signals for underwater communications are (1) stop—clenched fist; (2) go up—thumb up; (3) go down—thumb down; (4) go in that direction—forefinger pointing.

SEARCH PATTERNS

Line Sweep

1. Weighted buoy may be placed where object of the search was last seen on the surface.
2. Divers are stationed along line at points dependent on visibility.
3. After passing buoy marking object, the search pattern swings 180 degrees, pivoting on man in charge (or man at opposite end), and pass back through the area; repeat until the object is found or the search is called off.
4. The line sweep can also be used parallel to beach.
5. The line sweep may be used without actual line, if necessary.

Line Sweep (scuba)

1. Scuba divers may use compasses and watches to monitor time.
2. Guide swimmers signal by yanks on the line if the team gets off course.
3. Guide swimmers can determine scuba divers' positions by feel of line and observation of exhaust bubbles.

Circle Search Pattern (scuba)

In a circle search, if the object to be found is lying on flat, unobstructed bottom, divers may spread out just beyond the point at which they can see one another and drag the line on the bottom. Thus they should snag the object of their search.

Multiple Circle Search Pattern (scuba)

1. Use same method as described for single circle search.
2. Leave a marker buoy after each pattern to show area covered.
3. Overlap the pattern each time.

Parallel Search (scuba or free dive)

Drownings in bays or ponds usually take place near shore. This diagram shows the parallel pattern used in this situation. Notice that the man in charge may be walking or swimming in shallow water where he can see the bottom from the surface.

RECOVERY OF DEAD BODIES

How much time passes before a body is found after drowning— days, weeks, months, or longer—often depends upon currents, terrain, water depth, temperature, and clarity. Currents can carry a body for many miles along the shore, far from a drowning site. An example would be a person drowning in a large rip, pulled out from shore into a strong shore current, and carried miles before being deposited on the beach. One such example is a young boy who drowned in a flood control channel that emptied into the ocean near Los Angeles. The body was found weeks later near the Mexican border, approximately 140 miles away.

Various types of ocean conditions as well as land terrain in unpopulated places can hide a body for some time. Reefs or heavy kelp growths can prevent bodies that are underwater from moving. If the body decomposes sufficiently it will never surface, as would normally be the case when expanding interior gases cause it to float. A drowning in deep water—three atmospheres (sixty-six feet or more)—sometimes will prevent bodily gases from expanding due to excessive water pressure. If the victim wore heavy clothing, this effect will be intensified. Water temperature can speed up or delay the expansion of body gases. Warm water activates the bacteria that cause gas formation; cold water impedes their growth.

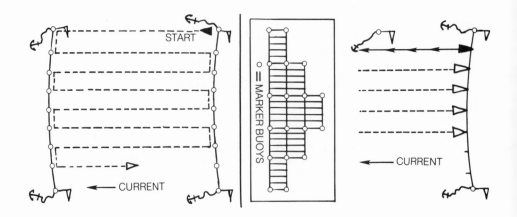

Parallel Search

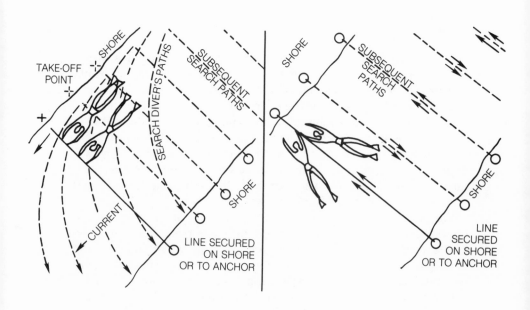

Line Sweep

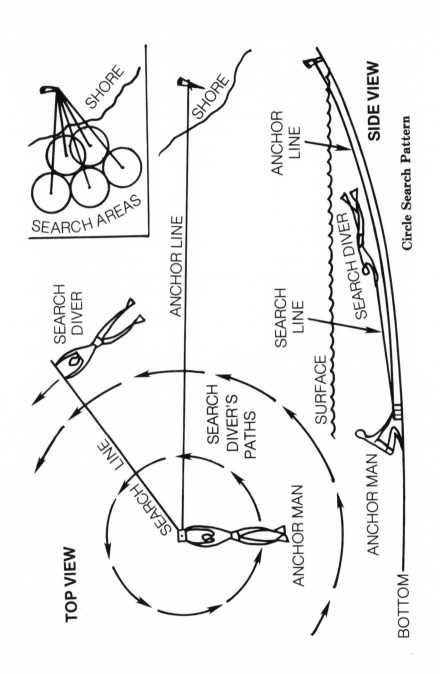

SHORE

SEARCH AREAS

SHORE

SEARCH DIVER

ANCHOR LINE

ANCHOR
LINE

SEARCH
LINE

SEARCH DIVER

SURFACE

SEARCH LINE

SEARCH
DIVER'S
PATHS

ANCHOR MAN

ANCHOR MAN

TOP VIEW

BOTTOM

SIDE VIEW

Circle Search Pattern

Handling a corpse over one-day old should be done with rubber gloves of a design that covers the forearms. Bacteria at work in a decomposing body could be the source of a serious infection, particularly around open wounds. Contact with any body fluids from the corpse should also be avoided.

After being brought to the beach, the corpse should be covered or placed into a body pouch—a leak-proof bag designed for this purpose. These pouches should be disposable; otherwise, they present a cleaning problem. Coverings are primarily to conceal the body from public view until the coroner or designated official takes over and also make body handling to be easier. Generally, a blanket used as a body covering should be destroyed if considerable decomposition has taken place. The coroner prefers that a recovered body be left as close to the discovery site as possible, taking care that an incoming tide will not disturb it.

Personal effects of the corpse should be left intact near the body. It is wise to contact officials involved in death investigations within the jurisdiction of the lifeguard agency. State laws vary related to corpse handling, and with foreknowledge of local procedures, details can proceed smoothly. Since arrival of the coroner or other official may be delayed, if state laws allow, a corpse may be moved to a nearby building. Otherwise, it may be necessary to stake off the area where the body lies to hold back spectators and leave one lifeguard at the site so that others can return to their posts.

Death investigators usually expect the lifeguard agency to provide the following information: (1) time victim was reported missing; (2) time victim was found; (3) what victim was doing prior to death; (4) condition of health and swimming capability, if known; (5) pertinent observations (for example, did victim strike his head on a surfboard or rocks, or collide with a boat); (6) were alcohol, drugs, or medication involved; (7) description and color of wearing apparel; (8) names and addresses of persons with the victim or witnesses to the ordeal; (9) next of kin; (10) the victim's age, name, address, occupation, or military status. Information taken at the time that the victim is first reported missing is probably the most important as it will aid prompt identification, notification of the victim's family, and proper evaluation of death.

Scuba deaths would, in addition, require a chemical check of scuba tank contents and inspection of other gear for possible malfunctions. Records should be kept of the type of gear used in any equipment-related death for comparison to other similar deaths. Eventual relationships in boating, surfing, swimming, and other accidents may be helpful in preventing future catastrophies.

8

Legal Ramifications of Lifeguarding

GENERAL PRINCIPLES

Although legal systems and specific laws vary from country to country and even from one state to another, it is crucial to the success of marine safety and ocean lifeguarding to know the legal framework and legal consequences of aquatic recreation. Even the most responsible agency or service may be called into court in a civil lawsuit or, on occasion, a criminal prosecution.

Many states have statutory provisions that make any beach or public bathing area owned and/or operated by a public entity immune to questions of liability. In other words, in many cases, the governmental unit may be immune from suit. However, this immunity is more of a guard against frivolous lawsuits than a mandate for carelessness. In any case, each jurisdiction should be checked as to how this issue is handled.

Those charged with the responsibility to administer the aquatic recreational areas must not be "negligent." Negligent conduct is that which falls below a standard established by the law for the protection of others against unreasonable risk or harm. The idea of risk necessarily involves a recognizable danger, based upon some knowledge of the existing facts and some reasonable belief that harm may follow. The capability of the person's conduct must be judged in the light of the possibilities apparent to him at the time and not by looking backward with "wisdom born of the event." The standard imposed is an external one, based upon what society demands of the individual rather than upon his own notions of what is proper. In the light of the recognizable risk, the conduct, to be negligent, must be reasonable.

The whole theory of negligency presupposes some uniform standard of behavior. The standard of conduct that the community demands must be an objective one, rather than the individual judgment, good or bad, of the particular actor; and it must be, so far as possible, the same for all persons, since the law can have no favorites. At the same time, the law must make proper allowance for the risk apparent to the actor, for his capacity to meet it, and for the circumstances under which he must act.

To reach a standard, the courts have created a fictitious person called the "reasonable man." All are held to the standard of what the reasonable man would do under the same or similar circumstances.

Thus, those engaged in marine safety must abide by the above and function consistent with those standards of reasonable care that have developed and are continuing to develop. Marine safety specialists and their administrators must act consistent with the "reasonable man" in their occupation. Hence, it is of crucial importance to keep current on practices and developments in the area of marine safety and administration.

A working knowledge of accepted and proven lifesaving techniques, equipment, and developments is of foremost importance. Worldwide information should be constantly exchanged and reviewed to insure practices consistent with what is proper or reasonable in the specific situation. This educational practice will help insure conduct consistent with what is "reasonable under the circumstances." Keeping informed and up-to-date will enable those involved in lifeguarding to better protect the public while protecting themselves against liability claims based on unreasonable conduct (negligence).

The parties who manage or administer marine safety and ocean lifeguard facilities can defend themselves best in court if they utilize methods and equipment consistent with what has proven useful and safe in other areas of the nation and world.

Those who undertake any work calling for a special skill are required not only to exercise reasonable care in what they do, but also to possess a standard minimum of special knowledge and ability. Thus, adequate training and practice programs are mandatory to avoid the possibility of liability for negligence. These programs should be continually reviewed and upgraded.

SPECIFIC DUTIES AND RESPONSIBILITIES

Where marine safety services are provided, adequate supervision and control are mandatory. It is expected that employees of the lifeguard system are properly trained to cope with the variety of situations that may be reasonably contemplated. This can even include the handling of drug and drunk cases on or about the aquatic area.

Any training program must be made consistent with changing times and circumstances. Marine safety services may entail paramedical aid and knowledge of crowd and even riot control principles. Thus, it may be necessary to expand training programs to include instruction from a variety of police, medical, and legal experts. In any case, it is important to be prepared for any situation that is reasonably contemplated. A training program should emphasize the legal danger in performing a function one is not trained for or performing in excess of one's training.

Since almost any incident where an injury results may initiate a lawsuit, certain procedural precautions should be established to process and record all such incidents. Also, procedures for transferring of the victim from the marine safety specialist to others must be established.

From time to time, there are situations in which, because of the severity of the accident, the police, fire department, or ambulance service may be required. It is a crucial part of the lifeguard's duty in drowning cases, for instance, to continue artificial respiration or to use the resuscitation equipment until the crisis has passed or qualified medical personnel have arrived and taken custody of the victim. In any emergency, lifesaving personnel must render immediate and temporary aid, where applicable, until proper professional help arrives. No lifeguard should ever assume the responsibility of deciding that rescue efforts are useless. If a hospital doctor arrives with the ambulance or a doctor arrives on the scene, the lifeguard should continue to administer treatment under the direction of the doctor, who immediately assumes legal responsibility for the case. The doctor or coroner will pronounce the victim dead or instruct the lifeguard to discontinue treatment; his decision is the legal and final one.

Procedures should be established for all crucial matters handled by those administering marine safety and lifeguard services. These practices should be incorporated into lifeguard training programs. In any incident, one should assume the worst from a legal point of view: It is always best to be prepared for the inevitable barrage of questions, especially from news media, and for the possible lawsuit that may result from the incident. The lifeguard and the operator should not attempt, by word or deed, to prejudge either the legal responsibility for an incident or its seriousness. In all cases involving any claim of injury, no matter how trivial it may seem and no matter how much the victim may protest "I'm all right," "It isn't serious," "Don't worry," or the like, the lifeguard should, at the first opportunity, make a complete report. This report should be complete, factual, and detailed and should be transmitted promptly.

The written report will be invaluable in providing a defense based on fact, freshly recalled after the incident, if a claim or lawsuit does result. Written reports, memoranda, and documentary material function as aids in litigation. They serve as a memory refresher at the time of trial and help perpetuate the truth during the course of litigation, which may extend several years after the incident. The lifeguard should never assume that the information is known to his supervisors. Personnel should be designated, preferably high ranking officers or administrators, as spokesmen for the department. The latter should keep informed as to all facts of important incidents as they arise.

Since it is impossible to cover the multitude and variety of fact situations that can result in legal problems, the following cases are merely a cross-section of what can occur. Some of the decisions in these cases would be different depending on the particular jurisdiction. Nevertheless, it is felt that the following will, in general, point out the issues that can arise and the way they are commonly handled by the courts. These cases can provide helpful guidelines, and the principles derived therefrom may be applied to similar situations.

CASE HISTORIES

The following cases indicate how a variety of factual situations can entail legal ramifications. Of course, in these cases, the damage has already been done, and the matter is in litigation. "Preventive law" should be practiced. Marine safety services should be conducted in a manner consistent with specific laws and the general standards of due care expected, so as to limit those situations and problems that give rise to litigation.

A large group of cases is concerned with allegations of dangerous conditions. In *Ide* vs. *St. Cloud,* a deep hole existed without warning or guard. Plaintiff's minor son was drowned. It was held that the city must give the same degree of care as would a private proprietor. In another case, seventy-five boys went swimming in a new area on the Potomac River before it was opened; hence, they were trespassers. One thirteen-year old boy drowned due to a sharp drop-off, which could not be seen from the surface of the water. No recovery was allowed. A twelve-year old boy drowned at a public bathing beach in *Mocha* v. *Cedar Rapids,* when he stepped into a hole; held, no recovery. In *Virovatz* vs. *Cudahy,* plaintiff's son drowned in a pond with an uneven bottom contour and depth with large step-offs and thick, heavy mud. No recovery was allowed.

In another case, an intake pipe reaching several hundred feet into Lake Michigan had been laid across the bathing beach. Next to the shore, for a distance of twenty-five to thirty feet, the trench has been filled in, and it appeared that by action of the waves it was also closed for a distance into the lake. However, about one hundred to one hundred twenty-five feet out, the trench had not been filled in and there was a hole some twelve to fifteen feet deep. At the point where the trench began, the water was three to three and one half-feet deep. Death of a twenty-three-year old young man was alleged to have been caused by the unguarded hole in relatively shallow water inasmuch as he could not swim. Plaintiff recovered, even though in Michigan a bathing beach is considered a governmental function, because the purpose for which the trench was dug was a proprietary function, providing the city with water.

Plaintiff's daughter drowned while wading on a public beach. The town had dredged some sand, creating a depression covering an area approximately one-half acre in extent and as deep as eleven feet. The girls were wading, could not swim, and had no idea the depression existed. Other people were in the water. There were no lifeguards or supervisory personnel and no warning of any type. It was held that the town should have warned users of impending danger.

In another case, a temporary storm drain ditch ran from the drain outlet to the beach over a new sand beach playground area. Often the ditch was blocked, causing an accumulation of water in a pool on the beach. Such had happened the morning the plaintiff's five-year old son was playing near the storm drain with three other children, all under five and a half years. The victim waded into the shallow end of the pool, and the water was soon up to his chest before he was noticed by the other children; he continued to sink until completely under. The lifeguard who recovered the body testified that the bottom of the pool was absolutely concave with solid sand, but yet muddy and murky enough so his feet could move into it. There was no hole in the bottom, but there was a bit of a step-off from the side of the pool. The blockage of the drain had been protested to city officials without results. Plaintiff was awarded $10,000 for the dangerous and defective condition maintained by the city.

In another case, a seven-year old drowned in a river located in a city park. The city was sued on the grounds that barriers and safety devices should have been used to keep the young lad from playing along the river, which had overhanging trees and excessive brush. The boy had fallen from an overhang.

Regarding concealed materials, a fifteen-year old boy dove from a platform in a lake maintained by the city and struck his head on a water pipe, which was concealed under water because of the coloring of the water. Lifeguards tried to keep people from diving in this area, and warning signs had been posted, but torn down. The boy suffered a fractured vertebra, which severed his spinal cord, causing paralysis. A few months later he died. Total recovered was $15,360. *Caporossi* v. *Atlantic City* also involved a water intake pipe. A twenty-four-year old man, honeymooning and not familiar with the area, dived in and hit a hidden pipe with injury resulting in his being a quadriplegic. He recovered $600,000 against the city.

In *St. John* vs. *St. Paul,* the plaintiff dived into a lake from a diving board placed about twenty feet above the surface of the water. As he struck the water, his head came in contact with a sharp object (not identified in the case) that cut a gash in his scalp. The water was clear enough that he should have been able to see an obstruction, and there was no recovery. The plaintiff in *Hoggard* vs. *Richmond* injured her left hand when it struck a barbed wire fence while swimming at a lake resort. It was alleged that the barbed wire was a dangerous instrumentality. Plaintiff recovered $5,000. In *Carta* vs. *Norwalk,* a boy diving from a raft struck his head on a concrete pier used to anchor the raft. The city had leased the bathing beach for operation; however, as lessor, it was held liable. In a similar case, *Jones* vs. *Atlantic*, a boy diving from a raft struck an undesignated object, breaking his nose. No recovery was allowed in this case; it was held to be a governmental function. In *Belt* vs. *Los Angeles,* an eleven-year old boy drowned when he fell off a groin, which extended across a public beach into the ocean. The groin was constructed to prevent the shifting of sand from the beach and not for recreational purposes. There were no lifeguards or warning signs posted. No recovery; not a defective condition.

Several cases are concerned with a depth too shallow for diving as a dangerous condition. In most all instances, the water was not clear enough to see the shallowness. In *Hoffman* vs. *Bristol,* the depth of the water under the end of the diving board in a pond was three to three and one half feet. Recovery was granted on the grounds of absolute nuisance. On a municipal beach, the water under the one diving board was eight to ten feet deep, while on the other side of the dock, the water depth under the board was only three to three and one half feet deep. There was no notice of such fact. A twenty-three-year old man severed his spinal cord, resulting in paralysis from the shoulders down, when he dived from a swinging diving device into the shallow water. The court found the depth of the water created an inherently dangerous condition of which the public was not warned. In *Caywood* vs. *Board of Commissions,* the "no swimming" sign had been removed and not replaced. A fourteen-year old boy dove into three to four-foot water, seriously injuring himself; $75,000 recovery was granted.

In *Hawk* vs. *Newport Beach,* a seventeen-year old boy went to a cove adjacent to the bathing beach where he dived from a rock eight feet above the water. He struck bottom, severely injuring himself. The city knew that some of the beach patrons for years had used this rock as a diving platform, but except for instructing its roving guards to warn of its dangers, did not provide other types of warning or regular guards. The city alleged that the rock could not constitute a dangerous condition because it was a natural condition unaltered by the city; however, the court indicated that a natural condition may give rise to a dangerous or defective condition, which needs attention by the city.

A pole that had been placed on the beach by city employees washed into the water by the surf. The injured plaintiff recovered. An old thirty-foot telephone pole, in *Benton* vs. *Santa Monica,* was being washed back and forth by the ocean waves when it struck the plaintiff. It was alleged that the city had sufficient time to remove debris, and recovery was allowed.

Plaintiff's son drowned when swimming on a Lake Michigan beach, due to the undertow. Plaintiff alleged that there was failure to warn of the dangerous condition and that the lifeguards did not have preservers and safety ropes available. Recovery allowed.

In *Augestine* vs. *Brant,* the town was held liable in a drowning for negligence in maintaining a public park and bathing beach on the shore of Lake Erie without giving warning of its dangerous character.

In *Feirn* vs. *Shorewood Hills,* a thirteen-year old girl slipped on the wet dock and injured herself. She alleged that the city was negligent in failure to treat the boards so as to prevent them from becoming water soaked and slippery and also in not providing a surface on the platform or some covering to prevent slipping.

In *Schneider* vs. *Lake George,* a fifteen-year old girl swam out from the dock about seventy-five feet and was floating with only her face visible above the water when she was struck and injured fatally by a motorboat, which moored in a city slip. It was alleged that the city was negligent for inviting both bathers and boaters to use the same area at the same time. Plaintiff recovered. In another case, an eighteen-year old died when struck by a motorboat propeller when swimming. The swimming area was not roped off in a state lake. There was no recovery; the boy was aware of the boat and, therefore, contributorily negligent according to the court's ruling.

In *Rafsky* v. *New York City,* the city was held liable when a child was struck by a horseshoe thrown by a lifeguard on duty. While the guard was acting outside the scope of his employment, the city had notice of such activity and was therefore liable. In another situation, when a fourteen-year old girl did not come up, another swimmer notified the lifeguard, who was in a boat in the middle of the lake, showing him the exact spot where the girl had gone down. The guard sent a young boy to try to locate the girl on the bank, thinking that she was not really in the water. After twenty minutes, the girl was found in the water and it was determined that had the lifeguard rescued her immediately on notification, she would have been saved. Thus, liability ensued. In *Pierce* vs. *Ravena,* it was alleged that the lifeguard was incompetent inasmuch as he had not acted immediately upon being told of the girl's peril and also that he had not complied with all requirements even though he had training and a Red Cross certification.

SPECIAL PROBLEMS

Special legal problems are most common to those areas that attract great numbers of people, even though the area is covered by a large and well-trained marine safety system. In managing such an area, local administrators should be aware of the controls they can achieve via use of local regulations (ordinances). For example, if surfboarding during peak swim hours becomes a hazard, same may be regulated by ordinance. The same may be true for problems created by dogs on the beach (which may be prohibited), diving off the pier (which can be regulated), littering, and use of alcoholic beverages. These and similar prohibitory and regulatory laws can be justified as a proper exercise of the police power, based on the authority to legislate for the "public welfare" and safety of the multitude.

Where a public beach is involved, is it legally feasible to close the ocean to the public? It most cases, closure of the ocean by those responsible for the safety of those using it when done pursuant to hazardous surf conditions, is justifiable, and no liability will accrue to the agency exercising its authority in this regard, assuming the decision is reasonable in light of all the circumstances.

Where dangerous conditions exist, such as a strong current or rip current, should warnings be tendered to the public? Generally, if those responsible have noticed said conditions, the public should be alerted. Of course, in view of the fact that those using the ocean can be "contributively negligent" in using same when hazardous, or in some cases deemed to have "assumed the risk," there are limits as to how much the supervising entity will be held to be responsible.

In a lifesaving program, the use of boats may entail certain aspects of marine or admirality law, which should be considered. Information in this area can be obtained from Coast Guard offices.

In popular beach or pool areas, consideration should be given to law enforcement and crowd problems. Deputization of those who serve as lifeguards may prove desirable.

CONCLUSION

Those involved in marine safety should not only be aware of the law, but should feel free to suggest changes in the law in accordance with marine safety practices. There are some specific laws that may prove unenforcible and hence impractical. On the other hand, there may be a need for new or revised laws to better enforce marine safety. These suggestions should be referred to the proper legal and legislative officials. Just as marine safety practices may change, so does the law. The law was not developed to harass those involved in the world of lifesaving, but rather to help guarantee the proper maintenance of lifesaving service. The goal of the courts and lifesaver are consistent—to achieve the greatest safety for the greatest number of those in or about our greatest recreational asset, the water.

APPENDIX: COMMON WATER SAFETY REGULATIONS

Every beach area, according to type of usage, terrain, and geological layout, will need certain regulations governing public activity to maintain health and safety. Listed below are most of the common beach and water regulations that are enforced at beaches and bays in the United States. They are usually written as state or municipal codes.

Beach Laws

Glass Containers—Prohibited

Broken glass in sand or shallow water is a hidden hazard for bare feet. Glass containers carried over slippery rocks can cause injury in a fall. The use of glass containers should be unlawful in public aquatic recreational areas. It shall be unlawful for persons to break glass upon any public gathering area, beach, sidewalk, and water.

Animals on the Beach—Prohibited and Exceptions

Persons should not be allowed to bring, leave, turn loose, or allow to go any animal on a public beach area. Animals, especially dogs, are unpredictable in crowds. They may bite, attack, or create general discomfort. Animal manure and urine are health hazards and uncomfortable to smell and step on.

Exceptions are Seeing Eye dogs in company of persons with defective eyesight. Beach areas set aside, posted, and designated as "dog exercise and training" areas.

Beach Games—Regulated

Games of sport and ball games should be discouraged in congested areas. Games with baseball bats and hard balls shall be prohibited or conducted in areas posted and designated for such purposes. All ball games or engagements in any sport should be conducted at such places and at such times as shall be designated for such purposes by the lifeguard department. Games of sport that are deemed dangerous, blanket throwing, and general rowdyism should be prohibited entirely.

Private Vehicles—Prohibited on Beaches

All vehicles should be kept off the beach and emergency ramps except emergency vehicles and vehicles that are approved by the lifeguard department. Exceptions are areas designated as boat-launching or beaching areas where a vehicle is being operated for the purpose of launching or beaching a boat.

Fires and Barbecues—Regulated

Fires and barbecues should be prevented in congested areas. Where fires are to be permitted, they shall be confined in fire rings provided. Barbecues on stands are easily knocked over by children at play. Therefore, they should be placed in the safest place possible, provided, however, that they or a similar device shall not burn park grass or other landscaping. Coals from a barbecue should be removed from the beach or deposited in an official fire circle. Fire circles should be used only to build beach fires for cooking or warmth. They should not be used as incinerators to burn rubbish and waste material, especially waste material that causes unpleasant odor or excess smoke. Fire rings should be placed in areas away from private homes or areas that could cause citizen complaint of fire hazard from wind-blown sparks. It should be unlawful for any person to abandon any fire without first having extinguished it. The ashes and coals, however, should not be covered by sand. Young children may inadvertently play in or step into an abandoned fire ring.

Waste Materials, Refuse—Prohibited

It shall be unlawful for any person to leave, discard, deposit, or throw away any can, waste food, garbage, night soil, vegetable or animal matter, papers, or any other refuse or rubbish upon any beach area or waterway. All waste materials should be deposited in trash cans or receptacles provided for that purpose.

It shall be unlawful for any person to move, molest, turn over, deface, or knock down any trash can or receptacle placed in any beach area by the lifeguard department.

It shall be unlawful for any person to throw, place, or leave any now dead animal, fish, shark, foul, or putrefying matter on any public beach or waterway.

It shall be unlawful for any person or vessel to pump, discharge, or dump onto any beach area or waterway oil, spirits, gasoline, distillate, petroleum products, or any inflammable material; or asphalt, coal, tar, bitumen, or other carbonaceous material or substance.

Fishing Spears—Regulated

It shall be unlawful for any person to carry a fishing speargun or similar instrument in a cocked or armed position on any public beach or public gathering area or within fifty feet of a swimmer in the water, or in any area where simmers are present. All spears, barbs, prongs, and similar implements shall be sheathed, covered, or removed. A speargun or similar instrument should be deemed cocked or armed unless it shall be in a harmless condition and incapable of projecting spears, barbs, or prongs.

Swimming, Scuba, Boardsurfing Instruction—Regulated

Swimming, scuba, boardsurfing, or other instruction in aquatic activities on a public beach or in a designated aquatic area by private enterprises that disrupts, creates general discomfort, or endangers the public on the beach or in the water should be prohibited. All private enterprise beach or aquatic instruction on a public beach should be conducted with written permission from the lifeguard department and at such places and times as shall be designated for such purposes by said department.

Overnight Camping—Regulated

Allowing overnight camping depends on various situations, especially sanitary facilities available. Most lifeguard departments and their governing agencies do not allow overnight camping except at designated areas with set rules and controls or upon special authorization for adult-supervised youth groups.

Beach Hours—Regulated

Hours that the public may use the beach are controlled by some lifeguard departments and local law enforcement agencies. This control is usually a result of a history of vandalism, crime, accidents, and residential complaint or for the purpose of cleaning the beach, which requires the use of heavy equipment. These beaches are usually closed during darkness or until the lifeguards are on duty.

Tampering with Lifeguard or other Beach Equipment or Facilities—Prohibited

It is unlawful for any person without lawful authority to deface, injure, knock down, climb on, break into, destroy, molest, or remove any sign, equipment, or warning signal placed for the purpose of safety on a public beach or adjacent water or any of the structures and buildings erected in a beach area by the lifeguard department.

Swimming Areas—Regulated

Only bathing and swimming shall be permitted in a designated bathing and swimming zone, and it shall be unlawful for any person to board surf in or to possess, control, or use a surfboard, boat, or any similar rigid inflexible device deemed dangerous by the lifeguard department to the other persons using a bathing or swimming area. It shall further be unlawful to permit said devices to be released, placed, carried, thrown, or discharged or to permit such devices to float, drift, or be carried into a bathing and swimming zone.

It shall be unlawful for any firm, person, or corporation to row, canoe, or sail a boat or operate a powerboat or any other similar device in the vicinity of and within one hundred feet of any bather or swimmer in the designated beach areas known primarily as bathing and swimming areas, except for the purpose of making a rescue or training of lifeguards.

It shall be unlawful for any person to bathe or swim in waters where warning signals have been placed except for the purpose of making a rescue.

Board Surfing Zones—Regulated

Only board surfing shall be permitted in a designated board-surfing zone, and it shall be unlawful for any person to engage in bathing and swimming activities, except such as may be incidental to board surfing in said zone or for lifeguards in training. It shall further be unlawful to operate, use, or play with any device that the lifeguard department deems dangerous to the user or other persons using said area. It shall be unlawful to permit said devices or any dangerous object to be released, carried, placed, thrown, or discharged or to permit such devices to float, drift, or be carried into a designated board-surfing zone.

It shall be unlawful for any firm, person, or corporation to operate a powerboat in the vicinity of or within one hundred feet of any person using a designated board-surfing zone except for the purpose of making a rescue.

It shall be unlawful for any person to board surf in an area where various signals have been placed.

Board Surfing—Controlled

Board surfing shall be permitted in a control zone except during the hours designated by the lifeguard department. It shall be unlawful for any person to board surf in, or to possess, control, or use a surfboard in, or to release or place a surfboard in, or to carry, throw, or discharge a surfboard into, or to permit a surfboard to float, drift, or be carried into a control zone during the hours prohibited by the lifeguard department, unless in the process of making a rescue or training lifeguards.

This regulation can be governed by a flag system or by posting permanent or temporary signs. Few swimmers and bathers use this type of zone at their own risk during the board-surfing hours.

Permanent hours may also be set by allowing the surfers to have the early morning or late hours or both and allowing the swimmers to use the area during the main part of the day. Surfboards prefer the early morning and late hours because of the usual absence of wind. Wind distorts the waves and either makes them unfavorable to ride or uncomfortable for the rider.

No Board-Surfing Zone

The following regulation is used in areas where certain surf breaks are dominated by body surfing use and are not designated as bathing and swimming zones. These types of areas will come into effect by public demand.

It shall be unlawful for any person to board surf in a NO BOARD-SURFING ZONE. It shall be unlawful for any person to board surf in, or to possess, control, or use a surfboard in, or to release or place a surfboard in, or to throw, carry, or discharge a surfboard in, or to permit a surfboard to float, drift, or be carried into a NO SURFBOARD ZONE, unless in the process of making a rescue or training lifeguards.

Surfboard Definitions

"Surfboard" shall mean any rigid, inflexible device upon which, or with the use or aid of which, a person can ride waves or be carried along or propelled by the action of waves.

"Board surfing" shall mean any activity that involves riding waves with the use or aid of a surfboard or being carried along or being propelled by the action of the waves with the use or aid of a surfboard. To "board surf" shall mean to do or engage in board surfing.

Closed Water Activity Zone

The following regulation may be applied as a buffer zone between designated permanent bathing and swimming zones and board-surfing zones. This will allow an area of drift for a loose or controlled surfboard in a wave. It can also be applied to any area deemed unsafe by the lifeguard department on a temporary or permanent basis.

It shall be unlawful for any person to board surf in or engage in bathing and swimming activities in a closed zone unless making a rescue or training lifeguards.

Bathing and Swimming Definitions

"Bathing and swimming" shall mean all bathing and swimming activities conducted in water except those activities that involve board surfing or those that involve the possession, control, or use of a surfboard or similar device.

Fish and Game Regulations

Lifeguards should be familiar with the fish and game regulations that govern their areas. The enforcement of these regulations should remain the direct responsibility of the fish and game department. Lifeguards may assist the fish and game department by reporting chronic violators or warning persons in violation.

Fishing Regulated in Aquatic Recreational Areas

It should be unlawful for any person to throw, heave, hurl, propel, or place any fish line with sinkers, sharp-pointed material, or hooks attached in or upon any public aquatic recreational gathering place deemed too congested with people by the lifeguard department.

Alcoholic Beverages

Different states, counties, and cities have laws that vary relative to the possession or consumption of alcoholic beverages in or on aquatic recreational areas. Most prohibit the possession or consumption therein or thereon.

Experience has proven that most persons under the influence of alcohol tend to create a nuisance to others using the beaches, resulting in police action and distraction to the lifeguards. They tend to get into serious trouble when in the water because they cannot think properly and are easily exhausted. On the beach in a hot sun, they are prone to sunstroke. A hot climate also speeds up the affect of the alcohol.

Scuba Diving Prohibited or Regulated in Official Designated Swim or Surfboarding Areas

Scuba diving should be prohibited in congested swim or surfboarding areas. The bulky, hard gear can cause injury to an unexpected bather or swimmer. In a surfboard area, both the diver and surfer can be injured if the diver unexpectedly surfaces in front of a moving board.

If a swim or board area is located so that it may block divers from a popular dive area, then an access could be marked off and marked as a "dive area" or "dive access." Such a marked area would prohibit normal bathing and swimming activities.

Refusal to Comply with Lawful Order of Lifeguard

It shall be unlawful for any person to refuse to follow or comply with any lawful order, signal, or other lawful direction of a lifeguard.

The key to this law is the word "lawful." This law needs supporting laws. Otherwise, in the courts, an order, signal, or direction by a lifeguard can be successfully challenged.

Air Guns, Sling Shots, Pointed Missiles, and So Forth Discharged, Propelled—Prohibited; Throwing of Sand—Prohibited

It shall be unlawful for any person to discharge any air gun or sling shot, or bean shooter, to throw, hurl, heave, or propel any sharp-pointed missile or dart, arrow, sand, or mud pie upon any public street, waterway, beach, sidewalk, or public gathering area.

Boat Launching or Retrieving—Regulated

It shall be unlawful for any person to launch any boat or similar device in or upon any beach area not designated for such purposes except for purposes of rescue or training lifeguards.

This law will prevent persons from launcing a vessel in a surf area where many persons are unaware of the dangers.

Floating Devices

It shall be unlawful to use any floating device in or upon any aquatic recreational area that jeopardizes the health and safety of the user or other persons.

This law can be used to control the use of bulky, dangerous floating devices in crowded aquatic recreational areas subject to dangerous surf conditions.

Boats Prohibited in the Surf Zone

It shall be unlawful for any person, firm, or corporation to purposely row, canoe, sailboat, or operate a powerboat or similar device inside any surf zone not designated for such purposes except for purposes of making a rescue or training lifeguards.

This law is designated to prevent accidents due to the power of a surf and to protect persons using a surf area for swimming, bathing, and surfboarding.

Diving or Jumping from Bridges, Piers, Structures, Land Masses— Prohibited

The general public should not be permitted to jump or dive from a public pier. This will prevent serious injury and a liable lawsuit against the pier owner.

It shall be unlawful to jump or dive from any pier, structure, rock, seawall, or land mass that is posted with a warning signal, sign, or direction of a lifeguard, except for the purpose of making a rescue or in the training of lifeguards.

Too many times, due to lack of skill or unseen underwater hazards, serious injury occurs to persons who jump or dive into the water from a height. If diving or jumping from a bridge, a boat may run over the person who is diving or jumping.

Digging Holes in the Sand, Building Sand Mounds or Castles— Regulated or Prohibited

It shall be unlawful to dig a hole in the sand that will endanger the person digging or others (sand is subject to cave-ins).

It shall further be unlawful to dig a hole or to build sand mounds or castles in areas frequently patrolled by lifeguard patrol vehicles or other official designated emergency vehicles. Any person who digs or causes to be dug any hole on the beach shall fill said hole before leaving the beach area.

Holes or mounds blocking a clear passage of emergency vehicles, especially during a call, are hazardous.

Sale of Merchandise, Goods, Property, and So Forth—Prohibited and Regulated

It shall be unlawful for any person, firm, or corporation to carry on any commercial operation or sell merchandise of any kind in an official aquatic recreational area or to beach or moor any vessel for the purpose of displaying it for sale on any beach or waters adjacent thereto, unless licensed to do so by the lifeguard department.

Delaying or Obstructing the Duties of a Lifeguard—Prohibited

It shall be unlawful to willingly resist, delay, or obstruct any lifeguard in the discharge, or attempt to discharge, of any duty of his position.

Abandoning of Vessels, Boats, or Similar Items—Prohibited

It shall be unlawful to abandon any vessel, boat, or similar item on any beach or waters adjacent thereto. A vessel, boat, or similar item shall be deemed abandoned if said object has not been removed seven days after an official notice has been sent to the owner of the item.

After official notice, any sunken or abandoned vessel, boat, water craft, raft, wharves, building, or other obstructions shall be subject to be removed, destroyed, sold, or otherwise disposed of by the lifeguard department at its discretion and at the expense of the owner or owners and without liability for said damage to owner or owners.

Weapons, Firearms—Prohibited

It shall be unlawful for any unauthorized person to carry, display, or fire any weapon, gun, or firearm on any beach or aquatic recreational area.

Changing of Clothing—Prohibited and Regulated

It shall be unlawful for any person to change clothing in or on any public beach area except at such places designated for such purposes.

Placing Dangerous Objects in the Water Area or Beach of any Aquatic Recreational Area or Public Beach—Prohibited

It shall be unlawful to throw, place, cast, hurl, heave, or deposit any glass, bottles, tin cans, solids, nails, structure rubbish, trash, or any article whatsoever that is or may become a menace to life or limb to any person in a water area or beach area that is public or designated as an aquatic recreational area.

Use of Mirrors or Reflectors of Sunlight—Prohibited

No person shall use a mirror, metal, glass, or any similar object in a manner that would cause the sun to reflect upon such mirror, metal, glass, or other object and interfere with the vision of any lifeguard or law enforcement official. It shall further be unlawful for any person to willfully reflect the sun from similar said objects in such a manner as to interfere with another person's vision on the beach or in the water.

Removal of Natural Sand, Rocks, or Vegetation from any Public Beach—Prohibited and Regulated

No person, firm, or corporation shall remove or cause to be removed from the beach any soil, sand, or rock without written permission of the lifeguard department.

Tents and Other Temporary Shelter or Structure—Regulated

It shall be unlawful for any person, firm, or corporation to erect, maintain, use, or occupy upon any public beach any temporary tent, lodge, shelter, or structure unless the said structure shall have two sides thereof open and unless there shall be an unobstructed view into such lodge, structure, shelter, or tent from the outside. A structure, lodge, shelter, or tent set up in this manner will discourage illegal activity by persons using them.

Engaging in Game, Play, or Water Sport Where Warning Signals Have Been Placed—Prohibited and Regulated

It shall be unlawful for any person to engage in game, play, or any activity on the beach or in or upon the water, to bathe, swim, surfboard ride, scuba dive, skin dive, row, canoe, or operate a sailboat, powerboat, or other device in areas that have been posted with warning signals, signs, or directions of a lifeguard.

This law will provide the lifeguard department authorization to stop any activity that may endanger anyone due to changing conditions such as heavy surf, cave-in, water or beach contamination, or dangerous marine animals.

Fireworks on Public Beach or Water—Prohibited

It shall be unlawful to light, set off, discharge, or have in one's possession fireworks in or on an aquatic recreational area or public beach.

Fireworks shall mean blank cartridges, toy cannons, toy canes, guns in which explosive are used, fire balloons (balloons of a type that have burning material of any kind attached thereto or that require fire underneath to propel them), firecrackers, torpedoes, sky rockets, Roman candles, "Dago" bombs, sparklers, or other fireworks of similar construction and any fireworks containing any combustible or explosive substance for the purpose of producing a visible or audible effect by combustion, explosion, deflagration, or detonation.

Electrical Outlet Use—Regulated

No person shall use any electrical outlet attached to any structure on a public beach without first obtaining written consent from the lifeguard department and paying such fees as may be prescribed.

False Alarms—Prohibited

It shall be unlawful for any person to purposely report a false situation for need of help to the lifeguard department or its employees. It shall be further unlawful for any person to cause a false rescue or call for help when it is not needed or to cause a lifeguard to enter the water upon a false rescue, leave his tower, or to have his attention drawn to a false alarm.

Laying Down Hazardous Objects, Surfboard, Paddleboards, and So Forth—Regulated

It shall be unlawful for any person to lay or cause to be laid any surfboard, paddle board, or similar object in a manner that it is against any lifeguard station or municipal structure or signposts or to lay down said objects in a manner that would delay or block the free passage of a person or vehicle.

This law will prevent such objects falling on persons or prevent persons from tripping or falling over such objects.

Climbing on Lifeguard Structures or Public Buildings—Prohibited

It shall be unlawful for any person to climb or cause someone to climb on any lifeguard station, ladder, pole, or public structure on a public beach unless told to do so in an emergency by a lifeguard.

Loud, Unusual Noises—Exceptions

It shall be unlawful for any person to make, continue, or cause to be made or continued within any recreational aquatic area any loud, unnecessary, or unusual noise that injures or endangers the health, the peace, or the safety of others, provided, however, that this section shall not in any way affect, restrict, or prohibit activities or noise by the lifeguard department or its employees who are in the act of performing the duties of their office, incidental to authorized repair or work done in or adjacent to any aquatic recreational area.

It shall further be unlawful for any person to use, imitate, or possess any directional sounding device used by the lifeguard department or its employees in or upon any beach area.

Disorderly or Offensive Conduct, Seditious Language—Prohibited

It shall be unlawful for any person to engage in any offensive or disorderly conduct in or upon any beach area, waterway, pier, sidewalk, or other public place, and it shall be unlawful for any person to make any loud noise or distrubance or use any loud, noisy, boisterous, vulger, or indecent language in said areas. It shall be further unlawful for any person in said areas to utter or use within the hearing of one or more persons any seditious language, words, or epithets or to address to another or utter in the presence of another any words, language, or expression or any seditious remarks having a tendency to breach of the public peace.

Unauthorized Wearing of Lifeguard Emblems, Insignias, and So Forth—Prohibited

It shall be unlawful for any person not authorized by the lifeguard department to wear or display any badge, uniform, emblem, insignias, or lettering designating said person to be a lifeguard in or on any aquatic recreational area.

Swimming, Paddling in Boat Traffic Areas—Prohibited

It shall be unlawful for any person to swim, play, skin dive, scuba dive, or maneuver any device without the aid of paddles, oars, a sail, or mechanical power into or on any boat channel or boat traffic area or lanes without the permission of the lifeguard department.

Hazardous Aquatic Activities, Endangering Others—Prohibited

It shall be unlawful for any person to use any surfboard, paddle board, belly board, skim board, ski, canoe, or similar device made of any hard substance in the water, beach, or surf zone in a manner that constitutes a hazard to himself or to any other person.

Pier Regulations

Motor Vehicles on Pier—Regulated

No unauthorized person may drive or cause to be driven any motor vehicle upon the pier. If authorized, the speed of said vehicle shall not be over five miles per hour.

Roller Skates, Skate Boards, Bicycles, or Similar Devices on Pier—Prohibited and Exceptions

It shall be unlawful for any person to ride or cause to be ridden upon the pier any roller skates, skate board, bicycle, animal, or any similar device that depends upon wheels for movement. Exceptions are handicapped persons in wheel chairs or similar devices, push carts, authorized motor vehicles, or maintenance carts or wagons.

Diving or Jumping from the Pier—Prohibited and Exceptions

It shall be unlawful for any person to dive or jump from the pier into the ocean unless making or attempting to make a rescue or training lifeguards. It shall be further unlawful for any person to cause another person to fall, dive, or jump from the pier into the ocean.

Water Activity in Area Around Pier—Regulated

Depending on geographical conditions, pier activities, pier structure, experience, or average surf conditions, control of water activity around the immediate water area of pier is regulated. Some governing bodies that have control of regulating the piers prohibit all or some aquatic activities to be conducted a certain distance from the pier. The average distance is usually 100 to 200 feet.

Sitting, Climbing on or across the Pier Railing—Prohibited

It shall be unlawful for any person to sit or to climb on or across the pier railing or to cause another person to climb on or across the pier railing except for the purpose of making or attempting a rescue on another person or training lifeguards.

Overhead Casting on Pier—Prohibited

It shall be unlawful for any person to cast any fishing line or pole overhead or allow any lure or hook to pass inboard of the pier railing while casting or hurling.

Cleaning of Fish on Pier—Regulated

It shall be unlawful for any person to clean any fish, crab, lobster, or shellfish except at locations provided for that purpose.

Trash, Refuse, Debris, or Disposal on Pier—Regulated

It shall be unlawful for any person to leave or deposit trash, refuse, debris, bait, or dead marine species on the pier or overboard the pier. All trash, refuse, debris, or unwanted marine species shall be deposited in a receptacle provided for such purpose.

Number of Fish Lines, Traps, and So Forth on Pier—Regulated

The number of fish lines, traps, or similar gear each person may use are usually regulated. The number of items used by each fisherman is arrived at by fish and game law, pier design, and attendance density.

Animals Allowed on the Pier—Regulated

It shall be unlawful for any person to permit any animal on the pier. Exceptions are natural fowl and seeing eye dogs when accompanying blind persons.

Fishing Spears or Guns on Pier—Prohibited

It shall be unlawful for any person to shoot, heave, or hurl a fish spear on the pier or into the water from the pier.

Boating Near Pier—Regulated

It shall be unlawful for any person to purposely navigate a boat within one hundred feet of the pier without written permission from the pier authority. Note: The distance may depend on a geographical condition, average surf, and the like, but one hundred feet is usually safe. A boat with an unskilled skipper can cause pier damage and entangle fish lines or endanger its occupants.

Fires on Pier—Prohibited

It shall be unlawful for any person on the pier to kindle or to maintain any fire or bonfire for any purpose whatsoever, whether in an open or closed container, brazier, hibachi pot, or otherwise, or to use any heating, cooking, or lighting device other than those provided by the pier facilities.

Trespassing on Restricted Portion of Pier—Prohibited

It shall be unlawful for any person to trespass or enter upon that portion of the pier restricted against public use by any order of the pier authority or to attempt to climb any fence or barricade separating such restricted portion of the pier from the part thereof to which the public is admitted.

Blocking Vehicle or Pedestrian Traffic on the Pier—Prohibited

It shall be unlawful for any person to block or delay any authorized motor vehicle or to obstruct or unreasonably interfere with the free passage of persons using the municipal pier.

Tampering with Electrical Pier Installation—Prohibited

It shall be unlawful for any person to break, destroy, demolish, deface, or in any manner tamper with any electric bulbs, light globes, light poles, light standards, lights, wiring, switchboards, switches, or other things constructed for or used in connection with the lighting of the pier.

Commercial Fishing or Trapping on Pier—Prohibited

Fishing or trapping of sea life for commercial purposes on the pier is prohibited.

Damaging of Pier Pilings—Prohibited

It shall be unlawful for any person to remove mussels, clams, barnacles, or other sea life from the pier piling with grab hooks or other objects that might cause injury to the piling.

Projecting Poles—Regulated

It shall be unlawful for any person to allow or permit any fishing pole to extend inward from the rail to a distance of more than four feet or to permit a fishing pole to block or delay the free passage of any person or vehicle.

Heavy Vehicles on Pier—Regulated

Every pier should have a maximum weight for vehicles and equipment posted at the entrance and a law enforcing the weight regulations.

General Laws Regarding Boat Launching from a Pier

Sale of Boat Tickets—Regulated

No person shall sell or offer for sale any tickets for transportation upon any boat of any kind whatsoever upon the pier, except from the space or office provided by the pier authority.

Boat Landing Time Limit—Regulated

No person in charge of any boat or other craft shall permit, cause, or allow such boat or other craft to stand or remain at any landing upon or near the pier for a longer period than fifteen minutes at any one time.

Control of Boat Landing—Regulated

The boat landing upon the pier shall be under the exclusive charge and control of the pier authority and shall not be raised or lowered by another person, unless by written consent of the pier chief authority.

Dragging or Rolling Boats, Boxes and So Forth over Deck of Pier—Regulated

No person shall drag or roll any boat, box, barrel, or other object or propel or transport the same over or upon the deck or other surface of the pier for a distance of more than ten feet or in any manner that defaces or damages the deck or structure.

Launching Boat Vehicle—Regulated

No vehicles or trailers shall remain on the pier for a longer period of time than is reasonably required to convey a boat to and from the hoist.

Common Boating Regulations

Water Craft Speed—Regulated

It shall be unlawful for any person, firm, or corporation to operate a boat, vessel, or other water craft at a speed greater than is reasonable or prudent upon any waterway that is congested with persons using such waterway for recreational purposes and in no event at a speed that endangers the safety of persons or property.

It shall be unlawful for any person, firm or corporation to operate a boat, vessel, or other power water craft at a speed greater than five miles per hour under the following conditions unless said vessel is in the process of making or attempting a rescue or pursuing a violator of law:

1. Between sunset and sunrise;
2. Within one hundred feet of a bather, swimmer, surfboarder, or any person who is in the water exercising an aquatic recreational activity;
3. Within one hundred feet of a boat, canoe, swim float or platform, or lifeline;
4. In a posted area; and
5. Under bridges.

Operating A Water Craft in a Reckless Manner or Under the Influence of Drugs or Alcohol—Prohibited

No person shall steer or operate a boat, vessel, or other water craft while under the influence of drugs or alcohol or in so reckless a manner as to indicate either a willful or wanton disregard for the safety of persons or property.

Water Skiing—Regulated

1. No water skier, aquaplaner, or free boarder and the towing boats thereof shall operate within one hundred feet of another boat, canoe, paddle board, float, swimmer, fisherman, or the beach except when taking off or landing in prescribed areas that are posted for such purposes.
2. In prescribed areas for water skiing, all motor boats shall adhere strictly to a counterclockwise pattern regardless of the number of boats in the area and shall be subject to the control and supervision of the authorized authority.

3. Operators of/or observers in motor boats shall signal with one arm in the air when a person or other hazardous object is in the water adjacent to or in the vicinity of their boat. Such person shall stop the motor completely when taking aboard any person from the water into the boat.
4. Water ski tow lines shall not exceed seventy-five feet in length.

Flashing Blue Lights, Sirens Used by Vessels—Regulated and Prohibited

No person shall shine a blue flashing light or sound, operate, or cause to be sounded or operated a siren on a vessel except an authorized crew aboard a fire boat, police boat, or lifeguard vessel performing the duties of their office. The sounding of a siren or a flashing blue light shall be a warning for all boats to beach or move to make a clearing and safe passage for a vessel showing a flashing blue light or sounding a siren or both. This section shall not preclude vessels from being provided with sound-producing devices as required by the appropriate Coast Guard regulations or the sounding of such devices in conditions appropriate for safety.

Towing Regulations

Any motor boat in the process of towing any object shall be manned by two persons—an operator and an observer. The operator shall watch ahead at all times. The observer shall watch the towed object and advise the operator of any hazard. The observer shall not be less than twelve years of age. Tow lines in congested areas shall not exceed seventy-five feet in length. Any vessel in the process of towing has the right of way and other vessels shall not overtake or follow at a distance of less than 200 feet.

Racing of Vessels—Regulated

It shall be unlawful for any person to conduct, operate, or take part in any boat race, demonstration, or exhibit of any kind with a vessel that interferes with the free use of any waterway or water area, unless a written permit for such event designating the prescribed area to be used and time of the event first has been procured from the authority of the waterway or water area.

Motorboat Mufflers—Regulated

Every water craft equipped with an internal combustion engine shall at all times be equipped with an adequate muffler in constant operation and properly maintained to prevent any excessive or unusual noise, and no such muffler or exhaust system shall be equipped with a cut-out, bypass, or similar item.

Launching or Removal of Vessels—Regulated

It shall be unlawful to launch or remove any vessel over any seawall, sidewalk, street end, or public or private property except at such locations designated for such purposes.

Excerpts from ABC's of California Boating Law

Motorboats are divided into the following classes:

Class A   Less than sixteen feet in length
Class 1   Sixteen feet and over, but less than twenty-six feet
Class 2   Twenty-six feet and over, but less than forty feet
Class 3 (a)   Forty feet and over, but less than sixty-five feet
Class 3 (b)   Sixty-five feet and over

The length of the motorboat is determined by measuring from end to end over the deck in a straight line, down the center.

Class A Motorboats Shall Carry the Following Equipment

1. One Coast Guard–approved life preserver, ring life buoy, and a buoyant vest, buoyant cushion, or other approved device for each person. If carrying passengers for hire, there are additional requirements.
2. A suitable sound-producing device when operating on coastal waters where international rules apply.
3. One fire extinguisher of approved type, with certain exceptions. If the vessel has spaces in which flammable vapors might collect, it should carry an extinguisher.
4. An approved carburetor backfire flame control system for inboard motors.
5. An effective muffling system for the exhaust of each internal combustion engine.
6. At least two ventilator ducts fitted with cowls for bilges and fuel tank compartment, if fuel used has a flashpoint of 110 degrees F or less, such as gasoline, and natural ventilation is inadequate to prevent accumulation of vapor.
7. Lights (under inland rules)
   a. One white light aft (on rear of vessel) to show all around the horizon (32 points or 360 degrees).
   b. One combined lantern on forepart of vessel, lower than the white light aft, showing green to starboard and red port, 10 points (112.5 degrees) on respective sides of the bow.

Class 1 Motorboats Shall Carry the Following Equipment

1. One Coast Guard–approved life preserver, ring life buoy, and a buoyant vest, buoyant cushion, or other approved device for each person. If carrying passengers for hire, there are additional requirements.
2. One whistle or other sound-producing mechanical appliance capable of producing a blast of two seconds or longer duration and audible for at least a half mile.
3. One fire extinguisher of approved type, with certain exceptions. If the vessel has spaces in which flammable vapors might collect, it should carry a fire extinguisher.
4. An approved carburetor backfire flame control system for inboard motors.
5. An effective muffling system for the exhaust of each internal combustion engine.
6. At least two ventilator ducts fitted with cowls for bilges and fuel tank

compartment, if fuel used has a flashpoint of 110 degrees F or less, such as gasoline, where natural ventilation is inadequate to prevent accumulation of vapor.

7. Lights (for inland waters)
   a. One white light aft to show all around the horizon (32 points or 360 degrees).
   b. One combined lantern on forepart of vessel, lower than white light aft, showing green to starboard and red to port, 10 points (112.5 degrees) on respective sides of the bow.

Class 2 Motorboats Shall Carry the Following Equipment

1. One Coast Guard–approved life preserver, ring life buoy, and a buoyant vest, buoyant cushion, or other approved device for each person. If carrying passengers for hire, there are additional requirements.
2. a. One whistle or other sound-producing mechanical appliance, hand or power operated, capable of producing a blast of two seconds or longer duration and audible for at least one mile.
   b. One bell.
   c. A fog horn is also required when operating on coastal waters where international rules apply.
3. Two hand portable fire extinguishers or one hand portable with fixed fire extinguishing system.
4. An approved carburetor backfire flame control system for inboard motors.
5. An effective muffling system for the exhaust of each internal combustion engine.
6. At least two ventilator ducts fitted with cowls for bilges and fuel tank compartment, if fuel used has flashpoint of 110 degrees F or less, such as gasoline, where natural ventilation is inadequate to prevent accumulation of vapor.
7. Lights (for inland waters)
   a. One white light as far forward as feasible to show an unbroken light of 20 points, with 10 points on each side of the vessel.
   b. One white light aft, to show all around the horizon (32 points) and higher than the white light forward.
   c. One red light on port side and one green light on starboard side (10 points each) with screen to prevent lights from being seen across the bow.

Class 3 Motorboats Shall Carry the Following Equipment

1. One Coast Guard–approved life preserver or ring life buoy for each person. If carrying passengers for hire, there are additional requirements.
2. a. One whistle or other sound-producing mechanical device, power operated, capable of producing a blast of two seconds or longer duration and audible for a distance of at least one mile.
3. Two or more fire extinguishers.
4. An approved carburetor backfire flame control system for inboard motors.
5. An effective muffling system for the exhaust of each internal combustion engine.

6. At least two ventilator ducts fitted with cowls for bilges and fuel tank compartment, if fuel used has flashpoint of 100 degrees F or less, such as gasoline, where natural ventilation is inadequate to prevent accumulation of vapor.
7. Lights (for inland waters)
    a. One white light as far forward as feasible to show an unbroken light of 20 points, with 10 points on each side of vessel.
    b. One white light aft, to show all around the horizon (32 points) and higher than the white light forward.
    c. One red light on the port side and one green light on the starboard side (10 points) with screen to prevent lights from being seen across the bow.

Sailing Vessels Shall Carry the Following Equipment

1. A fog horn
2. Lights (for inland waters)
    a. One white light of 12 points shining aft.
    b. One green light on starboard and one red light on port, each showing 10 points forward on respective sides of the bow.
    c. The law also provides that a small sailing vessel may carry a white light in lieu of the above to be shown temporarily when in danger of collision, but does not define "small." However, it is reasonable to presume that the size of a rowboat or smaller is intended.

Note: In addition to the above, sailing vessels should carry one Coast Guard–approved life preserver, ring life buoy, and a buoyant vest, buoyant cushion, or other approved device for each person.

Hand-propelled Vessels, Including Rowboats and Canoes, Should Carry the Following Equipment

1. One Coast Guard–approved life preserver, ring life buoy, and a buoyant vest, buoyant cushion, or other approved device for each person.
2. A lantern showing a white light, to be temporarily exhibited in sufficient time to prevent collision.
3. A suitable sound device.

Anchor Lights

Vessels under 150 feet in length when at anchor must show a white 32-point light forward. However, vessels at sixty-five feet or less, when anchored in a special anchoraged area, are not required to show a light.

9

Special Procedures and Functions

FORM AND REPORT WRITING

Efficient function of a department's equipment and facilities depends on the experience and knowledge of its personnel. And documentation, clearly and objectively recorded, is essential to assessment of a department's value.

The purpose of keeping records is to obtain facts that will form the basis of reports that in turn indicate the action to be taken by the administrative body in forming opinions about the operation. Accurate and complete records and report writing reveal in words and statistics a picture of most lifeguard problems and activities. Such records and reports should reflect the need for marine safety and lifeguard services and the effort of the lifeguard agency to provide the needed service. It is imperative, therefore, that all incidents reported to the service be promptly and correctly recorded for current reference and review and for subsequent analysis.

To be fully effective, a records system must (1) be comprehensive and include every incident; (2) be adequately indexed to permit ready reference; (3) be centralized to provide for adequate control and maximum utilization by clerical personnel; (4) be as simple as is possible, consistent with adequacy; and (5) lend itself to summarization and analysis to permit periodic appraisal of lifeguard services. Such a system will permit records, reports, and analysis to be used as significant tools of management, supervision, control, policymaking, and operation.

Without adequate records and reports, it would be nearly impossible to prepare and justify budget proposals. It is important to stress the keeping of daily records showing attendance, remedial actions, preventive actions, and personnel conditions for each twenty-four-hour period, along with space for bringing the month's statement up to date as well as for comparing the figures with those of the same month of the previous year. The monthly report is also of great importance to the administration for gauging the effectiveness of present services. It affords sufficient comparisons with other periods to point out significant trends and serves as a valuable aid to the director or chief, his staff, and division supervisors in evaluating the work of the force, planning new assignments, and directing attention toward areas deserving of greater patrol or surveillance.

Last, but certainly not least, is the annual report. Just as the daily and monthly reports are indispensable for studying lifeguard work over a relatively short period of time, the annual report is essential for analyzing department operations for the year. Furthermore, this report has the important function of informing citizens about their lifeguard department, in their capacity both as taxpayers and as persons whose cooperation must be secured for the effective execution of lifeguard work. In addition to the information already described as a necessary part of the daily and monthly report, the annual report will contain discussion and analysis of long-range departmental goals and objectives.

One very important reason for maintaining clear, concise, and accurate reports is the ever-present possibility of a lawsuit. Nothing could be more embarassing to the service that has done a good job at the scene of an emergency than to fail to file a good report, recording all known facts.

All accident and injury reports should be held in the files for a specified period of time designated by legal authorities. Reports are often used for important reference or evidence in lawsuits involving the sponsoring agency and/or individual personnel.

In all cases of serious injury or death, a supervisor will be present but may need help to collect important details, such as:

1. Names and addresses of all witnesses;
2. Written interpretation of the incident;
3. Witnesses' interpretation of the incident;
4. Exact time of incident;
5. Physical surroundings that have any bearing on the incident;

6. Presence or absence of signs and their exact locations; and
7. An estimate of the exact location of the incident.

Examples of different types of forms and reports used by marine safety and lifeguard services in the United States follow.

LOST AND FOUND ARTICLES

Marine safety and lifeguard services should provide a lost and found service as part of its service to the public. The following procedures are recommended for the depositing and recovery of lost articles. However, time limits and numerical values given may differ according to state and local laws. These procedures can be used as a general guideline and may be amended to meet specific needs of each lifeguard service.

Duties of the Tower Guard

When an item is turned in to a lifeguard tower, the guard on duty should:

1. Fill out a lost and found tag and attach it to the item (see illustration);
2. Call headquarters, where a log entry of the same information contained on the tag will be recorded; and
3. Notify area supervisor of items to be picked up at the end of the day.

Regardless of the article, all items will be tagged with all information possible.

Duties of the Area Supervisor

1. Pick up all lost and found articles at the end of each working day;
2. Place all articles in a large manilla envelope with the day's date marked on the outside;
3. Place envelope of the daily items in a safe storage place, such as a lockable filing cabinet;
4. If the item contains identification, try to make contact with the rightful owner;
5. Turn found articles over to the local authorities within the time limit required.

In most areas, local law enforcement agencies are responsible for the maintenance and disposition of any lost or recovered articles, and recovered articles must be turned over to said agency within twenty-four hours. Laws may vary, however, and local law enforcement agencies should be contacted prior to establishment of departmental policy.

CASE NO. _____
COPIES TO:

EMERGENCY REPORT

CLASSIFICATION						DATE OF OCCURRENCE	TIME OF OCCURRENCE	DATE OF THIS REPORT

LOCATION OF OCCURRENCE							DIVISION	

VICTIM'S NAME		SEX	AGE	DATE OF BIRTH / /	HEIGHT	WEIGHT	EYES	HAIR	DRIVERS LICENSE

ADDRESS	PHONE

EXTENT OF INJURY OR ILLNESS

CONDITION OF VICTIM UPON ARRIVAL

INFORMANT	AGE	ADDRESS	PHONE

DID AMBULANCE RESPOND?	VICTIM MOVED TO	MOVED BY WHOM

HOW OCCURRED

MATERIAL AND EQUIPMENT USED

SERVICE RENDERED

FURTHER DETAILS:

WITNESSES AND STATEMENTS ON REVERSE SIDE

EMPLOYEE IN CHARGE	REPORT MADE BY	APPROVED BY

CLIFF ACCIDENT ☐
SCUBA ACCIDENT ☐
WATER ACCIDENT ☐
BOAT ACCIDENT ☐
BEACH ACCIDENT ☐
SURFING ACCIDENT ☐
OTHER _____ ☐

SERIOUS INJURY REPORT
(For the Exclusive Use of the City Manager and City Attorney)

DATE _____ 19 _____

ARRIVAL TIME _____

TIME OF INCIDENT _____ TERMINATION TIME _____

HOW NOTIFIED _____

VICTIM'S NAME _____ AGE _____ FEMALE _____ MALE _____

PRINT   LAST   FIRST   MIDDLE

HOME ADDRESS _____ PHONE _____

CITY AND STATE _____

PLACE OF EMPLOYMENT _____

NEAREST RELATIVE _____ PHONE _____

NAME   ADDRESS

WITNESSES, IMPARTIAL   NAME   ADDRESS   AGE   PHONE

1. _____

2. _____

3. _____

4. _____

5. _____

LIFEGUARDS ON DUTY: YES ____ NO ____

NAMES OF DUTY LIFEGUARDS: _____

OTHER LIFEGUARDS RESPONDING TO INCIDENT: _____

NATURE OF INJURY: (Describe in detail) _____

LOCATION OF INCIDENT: (Be precise) _____

AREA: SWIMMING _____ SURFING _____ CONTROL _____ OPEN _____ CLOSED _____

EVIDENCE OF: DRINKING _____ DRUGS _____ NONE _____   AREA POSTED: YES _____ NO _____ HOW _____

INCIDENT: (Describe in detail) _____

FIRST AID RENDERED: (Describe) _____

EQUIPMENT USED AND NO. _____

OTHER RESPONDING AGENCIES _____

DISPOSITION OF VICTIM: POLICE PATROL CAR _____ POLICE AMBULANCE _____ COAST GUARD _____ OTHER _____

PROPERTY LOSS: (Describe) _____

NAME OF PERSON MAKING REPORT   BADGE   APPROVED   TITLE

NOTE: IF ADDITIONAL SPACE IS REQUIRED, PLEASE USE REVERSE SIDE OF THIS FORM.   CC: _____

WHAT OTHER REPORTS WERE MADE ON THIS INCIDENT?   NONE _____

DESCRIBE _____

9N-151 (10-75)

TYPE OF ACCIDENT:
CLIFF ☐
WATER ☐
BOAT ☐
BEACH ☐
SURFING ☐
OTHER _____

DEATH REPORT
LIFEGUARD SERVICE

USE ONLY IF DEATH IS DUE TO DROWNING

DATE _____ TIME OF INCIDENT _____
LOCATION OF INCIDENT: (BE PRECISE) _____
_____

SEARCH   START _____   YES ☐
TIME: FINISH _____   RECOVERY: NO ☐
RECOVERY: DATE _____   TIME: _____

VICTIM'S NAME _____   AGE _____ MALE ☐   FEMALE ☐
           (LAST)   (FIRST)   (MIDDLE)

VICTIM'S ADDRESS _____

DESCRIPTION OF VICTIM: HAIR _____ EYES _____ APPROX. WT. _____ lb. APPROX. HT. _____ ft. _____ in. RACE _____
         APPAREL: BATHSUIT ☐   WETSUIT ☐   SCUBA ☐   NUDE ☐   MAJ. APPAREL COLOR _____
                 CIVILIAN CLOTHING ☐   (DESCRIBE) _____

	NAME	ADDRESS	AGE	PHONE
NEXT OF KIN:				

WITNESSES:
1. _____
2. _____

GUARDED AREA: YES ☐   AREA POSTED: YES ☐   HOW _____
               NO ☐   NO ☐   _____
GUARDS ON DUTY: _____
_____

OTHER LIFEGUARDS RESPONDING: _____
_____

EQUIPMENT USED: _____

EVIDENCE OF: DRINKING ☐   DRUGS ☐   NONE ☐
APPARENT REASON FOR DEATH: _____

USE ONLY IF DEATH IS DUE TO DROWNING

SURF CONDITIONS:
    CALM ☐   SMALL (1-3 ft.) ☐
    MED (4-5 ft.) ☐   LARGE (6 ft) ☐
WATER VISIBILITY
    GOOD ☐   FAIR ☐   POOR ☐
WATER TEMP: _____
APPROX. WATER DEPTH: _____
TYPE OF BOTTOM:
    KELP ☐   REEF ☐   ROCK ☐   SAND ☐

INCIDENT: (DESCRIBE IN DETAIL) _____
_____
_____
_____
_____
_____
_____
_____
_____

MEDICAL AID RENDERED: (IF ANY) _____
_____

OTHER RESPONDING AGENCIES: POLICE DEPT. ☐   FIRE DEPT. ☐   COAST GUARD ☐   OTHER _____

NAME OF PERSON MAKING REPORT	BADGE	APPROVED		TITLE

WHAT OTHER REPORTS WERE MADE ON THIS INCIDENT: _____ NONE ☐   CC: _____
_____

DAMAGE REPORT

DATE: _____   [] PROPERTY
TIME: _____   [] EQUIPMENT
LOCATION: _____   [] UNIT - NO. _____

REPORT: _____
_____
_____
_____
_____

IS DAMAGE IN NEED OF IMMEDIATE REPAIR?   [] YES   [] NO
IS REPAIR NECESSARY FOR SAFE OPERATION? [] YES   [] NO

                                    REPORTED BY: _____

DISPOSITION: ASSIGNED TO: _____

[]   REPAIR DAMAGE IMMEDIATELY.
[]   REPAIR DAMAGE PER YOUR SCHEDULE.
[]   CHECK SITUATION AND REPORT BACK TO UNDERSIGNED.
[]   OTHER: _____

                                    ASSIGNED BY: _____

COMMENTS: _____
_____
_____
_____

REPLACEMENT PARTS: _____
_____
_____

WORK DONE BY: _____   TOTAL TIME: _____

REPAIR COMPLETED ON: _____   MATERIAL COSTS: _____

ORININAL COPY.........MAINTENANCE DIVISION
PINK COPY.............DIVISION RECORDS
CARD COPY.............ATTACHED TO DAMAGED ITEM

PERSONAL PROGRESS REPORT

EMPLOYEE_____ DIVISION_____

CLASSIFICATION_____ DATE_____ TIME_____

NATURE OF REPORT

[] COMMENDATION   [] REPRIMAND   [] DISCIPLINARY REPORT

DETAILS OF INCIDENT:_____

_____

_____

_____

_____

EMPLOYEES REMARKS:_____

_____

_____

_____

               SIGNATURE_____ DATE_____

DISPOSITION:_____

_____

_____

_____

_____

_____

REPORTED BY:_____ DIVISION_____

DIVISION SUPERVISOR:_____

DIVISION HEAD:_____

DIRECTOR:_____

CITY OF HUNTINGTON BEACH
HARBORS AND BEACHES DEPARTMENT
MONTHLY ACTIVITY REPORT

Month - Year

MARINE SAFETY STATISTICS

	THIS MONTH	YEAR TO DATE	THIS MO. LAST YR.	LAST YR TO DATE
ATTENDANCE				
Day				
City Beach				
County Beach				
Pier				
Night				
City Beach				
County Beach				
Pier				
RESCUES				
Swimmers				
Surfboarders				
SCUBA Divers				
Other				
PREVENTATIVE ACTIONS				
Boat Warnings				
Other				
FALSE ALARMS				
BOAT RESCUES				
Capsized				
Persons Aboard				
Vessel Value				
In Surfline				
Persons Aboard				
Vessel Value				
Fire				
Persons Aboard				
Vessel Value				
Other				
Persons Aboard				
Vessel Value				
MINOR MEDICAL AIDS				
Surfboard Injuries				
Head				
Other				
Jellyfish				
Burns				
Heat Exhaustion				
Other				

	THIS MONTH	YEAR TO DATE	THIS MO. LAST YR.	LAST YR. TO DATE
MAJOR MEDICAL AIDS				
Surfboard Injuries				
Head				
Other				
C.P.R.				
Immersion				
Heart Attack				
Overdose				
Resuscitation				
Immersion				
Heart Attack				
Overdose				
Inhalation				
Immersion				
Heart Attack				
Overdose				
Fractures				
Spinal				
Other				
Dislocations				
Heat Stroke				
Heat Exhaustion				
Burns				
Jellyfish				
Stingray				
Other				
AMBULANCE CASES				
Professional Services				
Lifeguard Emer. Unit				
LOST & FOUND ARTICLES				
MISSING PERSONS				
LOST & FOUND CHILDREN				
DROWNINGS/UNGUARDED AREA				
Swimmers				
From Vessels				
Surfboard Related				
DROWNINGS/GUARDED AREA				
Swimmers				
From Vessels				
Surfboard Related				

CITY OF HUNTINGTON BEACH
COMMUNITY SERVICES DEPARTMENT
MARINE SAFETY DIVISION
Weather & Surf Record

MONTH OF _____

DATE	WATER	AIR		SURF			WIND		ATMOS	VIS	BARO	ATTENDANCE
		HIGH	LOW	SIZE	SWELL	COND	DIR	VELO				
1												
2												
3												
4												
5												
6												
7												
8												
9												
10												
11												
12												
13												
14												
15												
16												
17												
18												
19												
20												
21												
22												
23												
24												
25												
26												
27												
28												
29												
30												
31												

CITY OF HUNTINGTON BEACH
COMMUNITY SERVISES DEPARTMENT

NEWS RELEASE

DATE: _____

RELEASED BY: _____

RESCUES	BOAT RESCUES	MAJOR F.A.	MINOR F.A.	LOST CHILDREN

FALSE ALARMS	BOAT ASSISTS	PUBLIC CONTACTS

NUMBER OF PERSONNEL: _____   ATTENDANCE: _____

WATER TEMPERATURE: _____ AIR TEMPERATURE: _____ SURF: _____

INFORMATION RELEASED: _____

_____

_____

_____

_____

_____

_____

_____

_____

_____

_____

_____

_____

_____

_____

CITY OF HUNTINGTON BEACH
HARBORS, BEACHES, RECREATION AND PARKS
DEPARTMENT

COPIES TO:

INCIDENT REPORT

CASE NO. **IR-** _____

NATURE OF INCIDENT			TIME & DATE OF OCCURRENCE	
LOCATION OF INCIDENT			DIVISION	
REPORTING PARTY	AGE	ADDRESS		PHONE
HOW INCIDENT OCCURRED				
FURTHER DETAILS				
EMPLOYEE(S) INVOLVED			JOB TITLE	
DISPOSITION				
REPORT MADE BY	REVIEWED BY	DATE	APPROVED BY	DATE

Log Entries

A log containing information on all found items should be kept in headquarters. This log should account for all items and aid owners trying to locate the lost articles (see illustration).

Log Book Entry

DATE: *5/1/81*   ITEM: *Wallet*

DESCRIPTION: *Brown wallet with ID*

WHERE FOUND: *Tower 3-Redondo*   LIFEGUARD: *S. Page*

FOUND BY: *John Doe*

ADDRESS: *123 Main St., Redondo Beach, CA*

POLICE STATION ITEM SENT TO: *Redondo Beach Police*

Report of Lost Article

When an item is reported lost, the following procedure should be followed:

1. Call headquarters and check to see if the item was found;
2. If the item was found, inform the individual which lifeguard or police station is holding the article;
3. If the item is not on record, inform the individual of the procedure for reporting his loss.

```
          LOST AND FOUND TAG

   Item: Wallet              Date Found: 5/1/81
   Description: Brown wallet with I.D.


   Where found: Tower #3 - Redondo Beach
   Lifeguard: S. Page

   Found by: John Doe
   Address: 123 Main St., Redondo Beach, CA
```

Any additional information may be written on reverse side of tag.

Information to Finders

Inform finders that if the owner does not claim item in ninety days, title generally passes to finder, who must claim the item directly from the property room of the local authorities. If the article is unwanted, the item may be sold at public auction or donated to a charitable organization. The time period of ninety days may be subject to laws governing that particular area.

KNOTS

The short list of knots described and illustrated in the following pages will meet all the ordinary lifeguarding situations. Guards must learn these knots and practice them until they can be tied with speed and certainty in the dark or when blindfolded. It is better to know these few knots expertly than to have superficial knowledge of a greater number.

A knot or splice is never as strong as the rope itself. The average efficiency of knots varies from 50 to 60 percent of the rope's strength. However, a well-made splice has about 85 to 95 percent of this strength. Splices, therefore, are preferred for heavy loads.

The strength of a rope is derived largely from the friction that exists between the individual fibers, yarn, and strands of which the rope is made. The twisting of these fibers into yarn, then into strands, and finally into cables is done in such a manner as to increase the amount and effectiveness of the friction between the rope elements.

Knot tying uses this same principle of friction. A simple knot, so tied that the strain on the rope adds to the knot's holding power, is better than a conglomeration of hitches, many of which serve no useful purpose. Usually the conglomeration of hitches has to be cut to free the rope from an object, whereas a simple knot could have been untied. Knots that can be tied and untied swiftly can make the difference between life and death or the saving and destruction of property.

The square or reef knot (Figure 1) is perhaps the most useful knot known. Do not use this knot to tie together lines of different sizes, as it will slip. The knot is used for tying light lines together, not for tying heavy hawsers. The square knot has one serious fault. It jams and is difficult to untie after being heavily stressed.

The sheet or becket bend (Figure 2) is used for tying two lines of different sizes together. It will not slip even if there are great differences in the size of the lines.

The bowline (Figure 3) will not slip, does not pinch or kink the rope as much as some other knots, and does not jam and become difficult to untie. This knot is the most useful and important knot for lifeguarding purposes. It is the most desirable knot for carrying heavy loads.

The clove hitch (Figure 4) is used for making line fast temporarily to a pile or bollard.

Whipping a rope end prevents raveling of the strands. Whipping is also useful at the end of a splice.

Figure 5 shows the correct method of making fast to a cleat: The half hitch that completes the fastening is taken with the free part of the line. The line can be freed without taking up slack in the standing parts.

Figure 6 shows the common incorrect method of making fast to a cleat: The half hitch is taken with the standing part of the line. Consequently, the line cannot be freed without taking up slack in the standing part. Accidents have been caused by the use of this type of fastening on the lines that must be freed quickly.

The fisherman's bend (Figure 7) also called the anchor bend, is handy for making fast to a buoy or spar or the ring of an anchor.

HOW TO SPLICE

Start the splice by unlaying the strands about six inches to a foot or more, depending on the size of the rope you are splicing. Now whip or tape the end of each strand to prevent unlaying while being handled.

Next form a loop in the rope by laying the end back along the standing part. Hold the standing part away from you in the left hand, loop toward you. The stranded end can be worked with the right hand.

The size of the loop is determined by the point where the opened strands are first tucked under the standing part of the rope (point X, Figure 8). If the splice is being made around a thimble, the rope is laid snugly in the thimble groove and point X will be at the tapered end of the thimble.

Now lay the three open strands across the standing part as shown in Figure 8, so that the center strand B lies over and directly along the standing part. Left-hand strand A leads off to the left, right-hand stand C to the right of the standing part.

Tucking of strand ends A, B, and C under the strands of the standing part is the next step. Start with the center strand B. Select the topmost strand 2 (Figure 9) of the standing part near point X

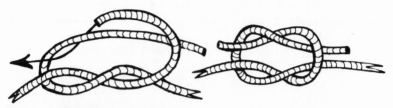

Figure 1. **Square or reef knot**

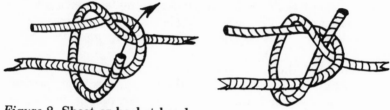

Figure 2. **Sheet or becket bend**

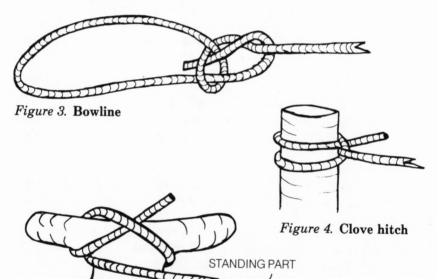

Figure 3. **Bowline**

Figure 4. **Clove hitch**

STANDING PART

Figure 5. **Correct method of making fast to a cleat**

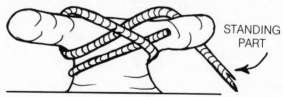

STANDING PART

Figure 6. **Incorrect method of making fast to a cleat**

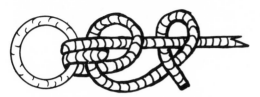

Figure 7. **Fisherman's bend**

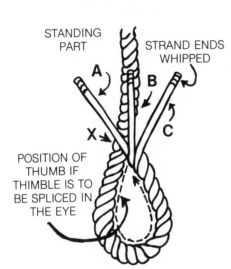

STANDING
PART

A

STRAND ENDS
WHIPPED

B

C

X

POSITION OF
THUMB IF
THIMBLE IS TO
BE SPLICED IN
THE EYE

Figure 8.

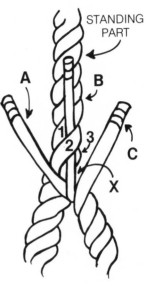

STANDING
PART

A

B

1
2 3

C

X

Figure 9.

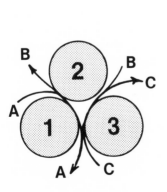

B

2

B

C

A

1

3

A

C

Figure 10.

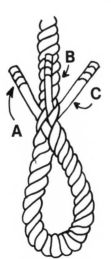

B

C

A

Figure 11.

and tuck B under it. Haul it up snugly but not so tight as to distort the natural lay of all strands. Note that the tuck is made from right to left, against the lay of the standing part.

Now take the left-hand strand A and tuck under strand 1, which lies to the left of strand 2. Be sure to tuck from right to left in every case.

The greatest risk of starting wrong is in the first tuck of strand C. It should go under strand 3 from right to left. Of course, strands 1, 2, and 3 are arranged symmetrically around the rope.

It may help to visualize this by referring to Figure 10, a cross-section through the rope at X, seen from below. If the first tuck of each of the strands, A, B and C, is correctly made, the splice at this point will look as shown in Figure 11.

The splice is completed by making at least three to four additional tucks with each of strands A, B and C. As each tuck is made, be sure it passes under one strand of the standing part, then over the standing part, then over the strand next above it, and so on, the tucked strand running against the lay of the strands of the standing part.

How to Make a Short Splice

A short splice is used where two ropes are to be permanently joined, provided they do not have to pass through the sheave hole of a block. The splice will be much stronger than any knot. The short splice enlarges the rope's diameter at the splice, so in cases where the spliced rope must pass through a sheave hole, a long splice should be used.

To start the short splice, unlay the strands of both rope ends for a short distance as described for the eye splice. Whip the six strand ends to prevent unlaying.

Next "marry" the ends so that the strands of each rope lie alternately between strands of the other as shown in Figure 12.

Working with either of the three free strands, splice into the other rope by tucking strands exactly as described for the eye splice, working over and under successive strands from right to left against the lay of the rope. Repeat, splicing the three remaining strands into the opposite rope.

Just as in the eye splice, the short splice can be tapered as desired by cutting out yarns from the strands after the first full tuck is made. After the splice is finished, roll it on the deck under foot to smooth it up, then put a strain on it, and finally cut off the projecting ends of the strands.

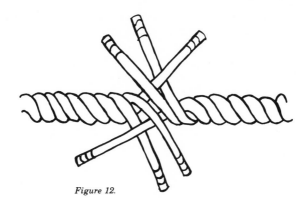

Figure 12.

JUNIOR LIFEGUARD PROGRAMS

Purpose

Junior lifeguard programs have been established on a communitywide basis for the express purpose of providing young people with an opportunity to acquire a sound aqautic background and become totally aware of the hazards of ocean swimming and other related environmental conditions.

The vast majority of programs are limited to young boys and girls between the ages of nine and sixteen. Because the course content demands above average swimming skills and endurance, it is strongly recommended that all applicants complete a one-hundred-yard pool swim in less than two minutes as a prerequisite. To stimulate interest and encourage continuing motivation, it is recommended that several levels of achievement be established and that written certificates be awarded for each category.

Personnel

Every effort should be made to have the program conducted by experienced ocean lifeguards of the highest caliber. As a basic practice of safe and sound management and supervision, it is recommended that no one instructor be responsible for more than twenty-five junior guards at any one time. It is also advised that when the program demands the incorporation of two or more instructors, a "head instructor" be appointed and delegated the role of chief authority. For larger programs of 200 to 300 participants or more, additional supervisory and/or administrative personnel may be needed, depending on the scope of activities and parent involvement.

Suggested Organization Classifications

Junior Lifeguard Program Coordinator

The program coordinator is responsible for coordinating and supervising the daily activities of the junior guard program. He assumes the position of direct supervisor for every instructor assigned to the program. Specific duties and responsibilities include:

1. Meets daily with all program instructors to discuss and outline the day's activities.
2. Meets weekly and at other necessary times with chief administrator in order to keep him constantly informed as to the progress of the program.
3. Evaluates the performance of every junior lifeguard instructor at least once annually.
4. Handles all parental communications within the scope of his authority.
5. Is responsible for scheduling, coordinating, and supervising all junior lifeguard special events.
6. Records daily and weekly program outlines.
7. Makes periodic inspections in the field to ascertain whether or not each task is being performed as outlined, checking whether regulations and procedures are being complied with, whether anticipated results are being realized, and whether available resources are being utilized to the best advantage and seeking additional resources if and when needed.
8. Reviews and follows up on all disciplinary reports filed on each junior guard.
9. Plans and reviews examinations.
10. Is responsible for all maintenance and upkeep of junior lifeguard facilities and equipment.
11. Acting upon the recommendations of the instructors, makes final decisions regarding group placements and rank promotions.
12. Maintains effective and harmonious relationships with junior lifeguard parents.

Junior Lifeguard Instructors

The Junior Lifeguard Instructors under supervision of the program coordinator are responsible for the daily training, discipline, and supervision of all junior guards assigned to their group. Instructors are expected to have the qualifications and to assume the duties and responsibilities as listed below:

1. Qualifications
   a. Minimum nineteen years of age;
   b. Minimum of two-years experience as ocean beach lifeguard;
   c. Basic understanding of the principles of educational psychology as it pertains to this age group; and
   d. Thorough knowledge of all phases of program criteria.
2. Duties and Responsibilities
   a. Meets with program coordinator and fellow instructors for daily and weekly program adjustments and evaluation where necessary.
   b. Meets with program coordinator for periodic evaluation of the program upon request.
   c. Meets with community organizations, service clubs, news services, and other agencies if participation is requested by the program coordinator.
   d. Maintains a soldierly bearing at all times and is a continuing influence of example.
   e. Is governed by the policy and objectives as established by the sponsoring agency and represents said agency in a manner befitting a public servant with a high degree of professionalism.

Junior Lifeguard Classifications

At the end of the first week of the program, all of the instructors should put into effect a placement and evaluation testing program for the purpose of grouping comparable abilities together in one of the four recommended basic groups. These groups are:

1. "AA" Total efficiency in all water activities, regardless of conditions.
2. "A" Efficient in all water activities, but Instructors should display caution when conditions are rough and/or swims are lengthy.
3. "B" Average ability to handle surf and wave size on a medium scale, and yet still on learning basis concerning surf hazards and conditions conducive to possible rescues.
4. "C" In learning stage of most activities surrounding the ocean environment. Careful training and teaching techniques to be utilized. Utmost caution should be displayed by the instructor and not forcing any individuals into any activities which they are not physically or emotionally ready for.

Junior Lifeguard Captain

Qualifications for junior lifeguard captain are:

1. Minimum of two-years experience in the program;
2. Must hold first lieutenant certificate and have an unblemished record;
3. Must test for this category the prior year in order to assume rank at the beginning of the following year's program.

Program Content

In order to maintain enthusiasm during any training process, it is recommended that a wide variety of activities be implemented. Those activities surrounding ocean lifeguarding are obviously most important but special activities must appeal to all. The instructor should bear the age level in mind in selecting from the following activities—ocean and beach safety, lifesaving techniques and procedures, body surfing, surf matting, surfboarding, volleyball, swimming development, first aid, competition in ocean lifeguard events, miscellaneous beach games and activities, field trips, and basic marine ecology.

For best results, the minimum recommended program length is eight weeks. This not only permits time for teaching and instruction, but also time to put that knowledge to basic use.

Depending on the size of program, it is usually best to divide the day into two sessions, with a break in the middle of the day for the instructor's preparation of activities. Five days a week with two three- to three-and-a-half-hour sessions for class time has proven effective.

Uniforms

Uniforms for both junior guards and instructors should be similar but distinguishable from uniform their agency employs. The junior guard uniform might thus be trunks, tee shirts, and in some instances, beanies of different colors to denote specific groups, categorized by water competence. The beanies are very beneficial to the instructor during a training swim since they permit him to pinpoint at a glance the exact location of every junior guard.

The departmental patch might be worn by the instructors so that the public can see that the program is sponsored and administrated by the agency. It is also recommended that the departmental agency insignia or patch be displayed by only lifeguards and that a different patch be designed for junior guard use, to make clear that junior guards are not employed lifeguards but participants in an educational program.

Notices to Parents

In order to alleviate problems of transportation for junior guards who live out of walking distance to the beach, it is recommended that during the registration period an address list be made up from all applicants' forms and made available to all junior guards and their parents. This permits a channel of communication between parents and aids in forming carpools.

Often times when a group of young boys and girls participate in a program of this sort, it is common for disputes to arise between junior guards that disrupt the class. For the occasional major problem requiring disciplinary action, use of a special form is recommended to advise the parent of the situation and of what action the instructor feels is necessary, whether it be a suspension for one or more days or expulsion from the program.

Equipment

Junior guard instruction should include equipment that ocean lifeguards use in their every day activities, including the rescue can buoy, lifeguard vehicles, and other equipment that can be made available for demonstration purposes at convenient times. Surfmats, surfboards, skin diving equipment may also be used, depending upon the aquatic ability of the group involved. Films and projectors are proven instruction aids for First Aid, rescue, resuscitation, or other related subjects. Marker buoys for competitions are a necessity and should be a bright, easily observed color.

Conditioning

Whenever physical output is required, it is most important to be conditioned gradually. A period of each session, preferably the beginning, should be set aside for exercising and warming up prior to any runs, swims, or the like. Following are some helpful warm-up exercises that all ages can easily perform. The number of repetitions should correlate with the age and condition of those participating.

1. Jumping jacks,
2. Running in place,
3. Arm circle back stretch,
4. Arm swing,
5. Windmill,
6. Burpies,
7. Trunk twister,
8. Cross-legged toe toucher,
9. Progressive toe touch,
10. Horizontal arm swing,
11. Leg stretch,
12. Alternate leg cross, and
13. Coordination exercises.

Discipline

Discipline is of major importance when one instructor is dealing with twenty to twenty-five boys and girls. It is imperative that order be maintained for the purpose of instruction. Signals are recommended for directing junior guards to return to a location, to fall in, or to get out of the water. Such a signal system may use the PA system, a whistle, and/or hand signals. Certain military commands also work well when the group is together with the instructor.

LIFEGUARD COMPETITION

The basic objectives of lifeguard competition should be (1) to sustain and uplift employee morale; (2) to stimulate personnel interest in rescue skill training; and (3) to acquaint the general public with water safety procedures and skills used daily by professional lifeguards to advance public safety at the beach.

At no time and in no way should competition or personnel participation in competition be permitted to interfere with established lifeguard operations or effective public safety at any water recreational facility.

Workouts during duty hours should be permitted only when they are part of an authorized, on-the-job training program or when taken by an individual during an authorized relief break. Workouts in a pool should be permitted only during an individual's off-duty hours without monetary compensation or compensatory time off.

Suggested competitive events might include the following:

1. 1000-meter open water or surf swim;
2. 900-meter run (300)–swim (300)–run (300);
3. 1000-meter paddle board race;
4. One-mile dory race;
5. 1200-meter iron man (400 meters each, swim, paddle, row);
6. 1000-surf ski race.

These events can be conducted on either an individual or team basis, or both. Competitors should wear identifying team beanies, and in the case of a surf dory race, helmets should be mandatory for the participants. Detailed instructions for conducting competitive lifeguard meets, including rules and regulations, format, and diagrams of the competition area can be obtained by writing the United States Lifesaving Association.

10

Principles of Organization and Management

OBJECTIVES AND GOALS

The primary objective of organization is to provide efficient direction and control of the marine safety lifeguard force so that departmental goals may be achieved in an easy, effective manner. All phases of service must be coordinated into one harmonious unit. From administrative to staff personnel and down through the ranks, all personnel should be provided with definite duties and assignments, and ample training programs should be instituted to insure that each man performs to his maximum capability.

ORGANIZATIONAL PHILOSOPHY

The responsibility for establishing the organizational structure for a lifeguard service lies with the head administrator of said organization. This task should not be undertaken, however, until the administrator (i.e., chief, director, manager) has made a thorough analysis of the individual needs of his service, based on the functions, responsibilities, and specialized services that his organization will be performing. If the operation runs smoothly and all personnel are provided with adequate workloads, the structure is basically sound. If, however, the workload of some employees is hampered or if there is low morale among the work force because of lack of incentive or communication, it is almost certainly due to flaws in the organizational structure.

CHAIN OF COMMAND AND SPAN OF CONTROL

It is imperative that tables of organization be drawn up in such a manner that each member of the work force knows exactly where he stands in the chain of command and to what individuals he is directly responsible. Supervisors and staff personnel should not be burdened with a span of control in excess of their physical capabilities.

All too frequently, the chief administrator will attempt to exercise a span of control beyond his capacity, and the end result is loss of control, ineffective direction, and poor communication. Since the number of lifeguards that can be effectively supervised by one man is dependent upon many variables, no set manpower ratio can be established. The number of men supervised is not so important as the physical locations of same, since the lifeguard supervisor can only be in one place at a time.

Depending on the size and scope of the services, the span of control should be such that the head administrator is not preoccupied with burdensome details of operations, thus allowing him adequate time to perform his primary administrative duties of planning, inspection, and a wide variety of management functions. Organizations that employ a large number of personnel and cover a vast geographical area should be subdivided into semi-independent divisions in order to insure a high level of service and adequate control of the work force.

The scope of any marine safety or lifeguard agency will usually be based on three vital factors—(1) geographical area; (2) extent of utilization by the public; and (3) financial condition of sponsoring agency. The number of personnel, especially those of permanent status, will vary greatly in direct relationship to the corresponding need for year-round service. For example, the majority of marine safety and lifeguard agencies throughout the United States and the world function primarily during the summer months. However, several agencies in southern California, Hawaii, and in various other parts of the world, since they are located in areas having a warm and desirable year-round climate, must provide year-round service. These services will generally operate with a small nucleus of highly qualified professional marine safety personnel and supplement their force with highly trained and skilled recurrent help throughout the year as conditions demand.

TABLES OF ORGANIZATION

Following are four progressive tables of organization that could be used as guidelines by almost any marine safety or lifeguard agency with only slight modifications. When organizing any size agency, the preservation of unity of command should be maintained whenever possible. Lifeguards who must answer to two or more supervisors will frequently be given conflicting orders, which more often than not creates a disharmony among members of the force and may even disrupt the effectiveness of a critical emergency operation.

Table I. Minimal Operation

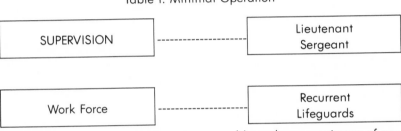

SUPERVISION	Lieutenant Sergeant
Work Force	Recurrent Lifeguards

Off season: In most instances, would employ a maximum of one or two permanent employees. Quite possibly would not employ any full-time personnel. (It is recommended that any year-round operation employ a minimum of two permanent personnel in order to provide backup for critical rescues and to compensate for days off, vacations, sick leave, and relief breaks.)

Summer season: Ten to fifteen, recurrent. Even when size of service is extremely small, a minimum of two supervisors should be employed to provide a maximum daily control of work forces.

Note: Although financing is often extremely influential, one-man coverage should be avoided whenever possible because of the following disadvantages—(1) provides no backup for critical emergencies; (2) when guard is making a rescue, swimming area is left unprotected; (3) relief opportunity is negated.

If a two- or three-man staff is employed, these problems will be virtually nonexistent. However, one of the guards should be put in charge, in order to maintain control and delegate responsibility for making emergency decisions to one man.

Table II. Moderate Operation

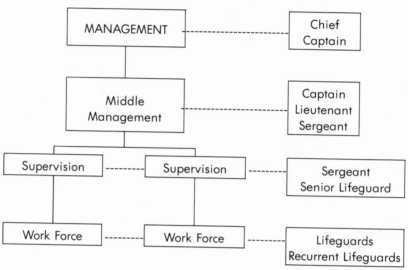

Off season: Year-round service in almost all instances. employs two to five permanent personnel. Management position almost entirely administrative.

Summer season: Fifteen to fifty recurrent lifeguards. Due to size of force and scope of operation, responsibility is subdivided in order to provide sufficient backup and supervisory control.

RECOMMENDED LIFEGUARD CLASSIFICATIONS

Although no two lifeguard or marine safety organizations are the same, the following job classifications, with slight modifications, would fit the needs of almost any marine safety lifeguard operation. It should be pointed out, however, that the classifications are based on major operations, and in the case of a relatively small operation, significant changes would have to be made depending on what titles were to be utilized.

These classifications represent the ultimate in the marine safety and/or lifeguard profession. While it would be superfluous to assume that every marine safety or lifeguard agency could establish their organization at this level, it is strongly recommended that agencies set their goals accordingly and continually strive to achieve that which is considered maximum. The stereotype lifeguard of the "ukulele days" has long since vanished from the scene, although a considerable segment of the public is still unaware of this fact. Every

Table III. Major Operation

| MANAGEMENT | ---------- | Director
Chief
Assistant Director
Captain |

Middle Management	--	Middle Management	--	Middle Management	--	Captain Lieutenant
Supervision	--	Supervision	--	Supervision	--	Lieutenant Sergeant Senior Guard
Work Force	--	Work Force	--	Work Force	--	Senior Guards Rescue Boat Operator Lifeguards Recurrent Lifeguards

Off season: Minimum of ten to fifteen permanent personnel. Large-scale operation. Administrative, middle management, and division supervisors are all permanent personnel.

Summer season: Minimum of fifty or more recurrent personnel. Areas are vast and heavily populated, so they are subdivided into semi-independent operating divisions, each division being divided into two or more areas. Most major operations will supplement their coverage with two or more ocean rescue vessels.

---

lifeguard, regardless of the size of his service or the nature and scope of his duties and responsibilities, should be encouraged to represent himself in a manner worthy of the profession.

Director of Marine Safety

Under direction from the governing body or chief administrator, the director shall plan, organize, direct, and control operations of a marine safety service and do related work as required.

Table IV. Total Marine Operation

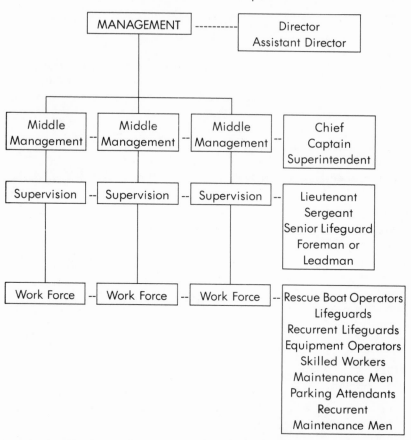

Off season:	Large-scale year-round operation. Minimum of twenty-five persons permanently employed. Several independent functions performed under the direction of one administrative body.
Summer season:	Based on minimum supplement of one hundred recurrent employees.

Note: Many lifeguard services operate as a semi-independent function of a recreation department. While this practice works well when in conjunction with pool operations, it is not generally advisable to coordinate surf beach operations with recreation activities, unless the administrative staff has a marine safety background. Public safety per se is not a primary function of a recreation department, and where possible, this type of joint service should be avoided.

Typical Tasks

The director of marine safety plans, organizes, directs, and controls all phases of the operation and coordinates activities of a marine safety service; formulates and directs the implementation of operating policies; prepares and administers budgets; interviews, hires, reviews the work of, and evaluates personnel; plans and supervises development of beach and harbor properties; directs and administers lease agreements between his governmental agency and all commercial businesses operating within the boundaries of his jurisdiction; plans, evaluates, and directs the operation and development of beach parking facilities; is involved in the development of harbors, waterways, beaches, and piers; reviews the performance of safety and rescue operations; coordinates these operations with other agencies; directs through subordinates the maintenance and repair of all boats, vehicles, and equipment; represents his service at hearings affecting his service and the governing body; assists in drafting proposed legislation; speaks before public groups interested in departmental activities; directs a program of public relations; directs the training activities for personnel; is subject to emergency call; represents his service at general meetings of the governing body and at special meetings as required; and is responsible for marine safety protection in general.

Employment Standards

- High school graduate or G.E.D.;
- Four-years experience in the field of aquatics and marine safety;
- Four years of college or four years in a responsible administrative capacity exercising management control over an assigned function or department, including responsibility for the supervision of personnel and budgetary controls.

Knowledge Of

- Basic oceanography and marine science;
- Principles of organization and management, including budgetary, personnel, and public relation practices
- Basic principles of marine safety administration and lifesaving operations and of ecological problems relative to areas of responsibility.

Ability To

- Plan, organize, and direct the activities of employees performing a variety of functions;
- Interpret, explain, and enforce harbor, beach, and pier laws, ordinances, rules, and regulations;

- Establish and maintain effective relationships with persons and agencies concerned with the department;
- Speak before public groups;
- Prepare and review reports and the maintenance of records;
- Represent governing body on their behalf in those matters pertaining to beach and harbor development and operation which involve federal, state, and/or county negotiation.

Assistant Director of Marine Safety

Definition

The assistant director of marine safety directs and supervises the activities of the various divisions within the service; makes recommendations in terms of personnel, apparatus, equipment, and future development; works in close communication with the director, keeping him advised of daily activities and progress of the department; makes recommendations concerning the development of ordinances, laws, and regulations regarding the harbor, beaches, pier, and parking lots; submits monthly and annual reports; directs the maintenance of departmental records; prepares departmental budget estimates; sets up guidelines of operation for departmental training and scheduling of personnel; reviews and approves departmental reports; coordinates departmental safety programs; supervises and controls departmental expenditures; interviews, reviews work of, evaluates, and hires the majority of departmental supervisory personnel; controls and supervises the issuance of the various beach, pier, and parking lot permits; and is responsible for marine safety protection.

Employment Standards

- High school graduate or G.E.D.;
- Four-years experience in the field of aquatics and marine safety;
- Four years of college or four years in a responsible administrative capacity exercising management control over an assigned function or department, including the responsibility for the supervision of personnel and the exercise of budgetary controls.

Knowledge Of

- Basic oceanography and marine science;
- Principles of organization and management, including budgetary, personnel, and public relations practices;
- Basic principles of marine safety administration and lifesaving operations;
- Functions performed and services provided by all departmental divisions and ecological problems relative to area of responsibility.

Ability To

- Plan, organize, and direct the activities of employees performing a variety of duties;
- Interpret, explain, and enforce harbor, beach, and pier laws, ordinances, rules, and regulations;
- Establish and maintain effective relationships with persons and agencies concerned with his service;
- Prepare and review reports and maintain records;
- Speak before large public groups;
- Maintain discipline and evaluate the performance of subordinate personnel.

Marine Safety Chief

Definition

Under administrative direction, plans, organizes, directs, and controls the operation of an accredited marine safety agency.

Typical Tasks

- Formulates and directs the implementation of operational policies;
- Prepares and administers budgets;
- Directs, through subordinates, the enforcement of traffic and safety regulations in the usage of those water recreational areas under the jurisdiction of his service;
- Reviews the performance of safety and rescue operations and coordinates same with other agencies as required;
- Directs training activities for all personnel;
- Represents his service at legislative and other meetings affecting the interests of his service and/or governmental agencies;
- Establishes a program of public relations;
- Is subject to twenty-four-hour emergency call;
- Makes frequent critical decisions involving life and death emergencies;
- Represents his service at all meetings of the governing body of his department;
- Is responsible for marine safety protection.

Employment Standards

- High school graduate or G.E.D.;
- Five-years experience in the field of marine safety, three of which have been relative to ocean lifeguarding;
- Four years of college and/or four years in a responsible administrative capacity, exercising management control over an assigned function or department, including the responsibility for the supervision of personnel and exercise of budgetary controls.

Knowledge Of

- Principles of organization and management, including budgetary, personnel, and public relations practices;
- Basic principles of marine safety administration and lifesaving operations;
- All functions and duties performed by the service;
- Basic oceanography;
- Ecological problems relative to his areas of responsibility.

Ability To

- Plan, organize, and direct activities of employees performing a variety of functions;
- Interpret, explain, and enforce relative laws, ordinances, and regulations;
- Establish and maintain effective relationships with persons and agencies concerned with his service;
- Speak before large public groups;
- Prepare and review reports and maintain records;
- Represent service on behalf of governing body in matters pertaining to beach and harbor development and operation involving federal, state, and/or county negotiation;
- Plan, develop, and coordinate regional water recreational developments and facilities.

Marine Safety Captain

Definition

Subject to the determination of policy as set forth by the lifeguard chief, plans, directs, supervises, and reviews the operation and activities of an accredited ocean lifeguard agency and does related work as required.

Typical Tasks

The marine safety captain directs and supervises the activities of the various divisions within the department; makes recommendations in terms of personnel, apparatus, equipment, and future development; works in close communication with the lifeguard chief or next ranking superior, keeping him advised daily of the activities and progress of the service; makes recommendations concerning the development of ordinances, laws, and regulations; submits monthly and annual reports; directs the maintenance of records; prepares preliminary budget estimates, sets up guidelines of operation for training and scheduling of personnel; reviews and approves reports; coordinates safety programs; supervises and controls disciplinary policies and procedures; is subject to twenty-four-hour emergency call; responds to emergency calls when off duty; directs, supervises, and controls departmental expenditures; interviews, reviews the work of, evaluates, and hires the majority of personnel; and is responsible for marine safety protection.

Employment Standards

- High school graduate or G.E.D.;
- Four-years experience in the field of marine safety;
- Four years of college or four years in a responsible administrative capacity exercising management control over an assigned function, division, or department, including the responsibility for the supervision of personnel and the exercise of budgetary control;
- Valid first aid instructor's certificate issued by the American Red Cross Association or emergency medical technician—I rating;
- Valid drivers license;
- Scuba certification from recognized authority;
- Cardio-pulmonary resuscitation instructor's certification from recognized authority.

Knowledge Of

- Principles of organization and management, including budgetary, personnel, and public relation practices;
- Basic principles of marine safety administration and supervision;
- Functions and service performed by all divisions;
- Principles, practices, and concepts of modern lifesaving techniques, of small craft, harbor, and boating safety, and of equipment and apparatus used;
- First aid practices and principles, including highly specialized paramedical techniques;
- All rules and regulations and applicable laws and ordinances;
- Basic law enforcement practices dealing with the laws of arrest and search and seizure;
- Basic oceanography;
- Principles and practices of underwater search and recovery techniques;
- Basic principles and techniques used in systematic filing of records;
- Marine law, regulations, and rules of the road.

Ability To

- Plan, organize, and direct the activities of employees performing a variety of functions;
- Interpret, explain, and enforce relative laws, ordinances, regulations, and basic law enforcement practices dealing with the laws of arrest, and search and seizure;
- Establish and maintain effective relationships with concerned persons and agencies;
- Prepare and review reports and maintain records;
- Speak before large public groups;

- Maintain discipline and evaluate the performance of subordinate personnel;
- Evaluate emergency situations and adopt effective courses of action;
- Maintain an effective communication system.

Marine Safety Lieutenant

Definition

Under supervision, supervises and coordinates the activities and operations of his assigned division and does related work as required.

Typical Tasks

The marine safety lieutenant plans, coordinates, supervises, and reviews all activities of his division, including those relating to personnel, vehicle, and boat operations and the maintenance of an effective communications system; makes recommendations in matters of personnel, apparatus, and equipment; supervises and coordinates the daily maintenance and operation of public relations and education functions relative to his division; plans and prepares examinations and training programs; prepares budget estimates; submits monthly and annual reports; sets up schedules of operations; supervises the training for new personnel; receives and gives interviews to the public on the activities of his division; gives lectures to educational institutions, civic clubs, and paramedical organizations; reviews reports; follows up on major emergencies; is subject to twenty-four-hour emergency call; responds to emergencies when off duty; represents department at various lifesaving, first aid, and water safety programs; coordinates and supervises law enforcement program; evaluates the overall job performance of personnel; makes frequent critical decisions involving life and death emergencies; operates specialized lifesaving equipment and performs various paramedical first aid practices of a highly skilled nature, and is responsible for marine safety protection.

Employment Standards

- High school graduate or G.E.D.;
- Four-years experience as an ocean lifeguard;
- Two years of college or four years in a responsible supervisory and/or administrative capacity, exercising control over an assigned function or area, including the responsibility for the supervision of personnel and the exercise of basic budgetary functions;
- Valid first aid instructor's certificate issued by American Red Cross Association or emergency medical technician—1 rating.

- Valid drivers license; National Surf Life Saving Association certification in supervising and lifeguarding;
- Scuba certification from recognized authority;
- Cardio-pulmonary resuscitation certificate from recogized authority.

Knowledge Of

- Principles and practices of modern lifesaving techniques, of small craft, harbor and boating safety, and of equipment and apparatus used;
- First aid practices and principles, including highly specialized paramedical techniques;
- Rules and regulations and applicable laws and ordinances;
- Basic law enforcement practices dealing with the laws of arrest, and search and seizure;
- Principles of organization and management including budgetary, personnel, and public relations practices;
- Principles and practices of underwater search and recovery techniques and basic diving physics;
- Basic principles and techniques of systematic filing of records and logs;
- Basic operation of all other departmental divisions;
- Marine law, regulations, and rules of the road.

Ability To

- Plan, organize, and supervise the activities of an assigned division;
- Plan and organize training programs;
- Maintain outstanding public relations and services;
- Interpret and explain relative laws, ordinances, regulations, rules of the road, and basic law enforcement practices dealing with the laws of arrest and search and seizure;
- Prepare clear and concise reports and review reports of subordinate personnel;
- Maintain discipline and evaluate the performance of subordinate personnel;
- Size up emergency situations and adopt effective courses of action;
- Speak before large public groups;
- Maintain effective relationships with other persons and agencies.

Marine Safety Sergeant

Definition

Under direction, coordinates and supervises the activities of his assigned area and does related work as required.

Typical Tasks

The marine safety sergeant supervises and coordinates the daily activities and operation in his assigned area; plans and coordinates schedules of operation; patrols his area periodically, making sure that all personnel are alert, and that activities are in order; assumes charge of all major emergencies until relieved by a superior officer; is responsible for the maintenance of equipment, facilities, and supplies; supervises and coordinates training drills; answers questions and assists the public; coordinates and directs underwater rescue operations; maintains personnel discipline; is subject to twenty-four-hour emergency call; operates specialized lifesaving and fire-fighting equipment and performs various paramedical first aid practices; represents department at various lifesaving, first aid, and water safety programs and clinics; evaluates the overall job performances of subordinate personnel; gives lectures to various educational supervisors in the exercise of basic budgetary functions; and is responsible for marine safety protection.

Employment Standards

- High school graduate or G.E.D.;
- Two-years experience as ocean lifeguard;
- Valid first aid instructor's certificate issued by American Red Cross Association or emergency medical technician—1 rating;
- Minimum age, twenty-one years;
- Valid drivers license;
- Scuba certification from recognized authority;
- Cardio-pulmonary resuscitation instructor's certificate from recognized authority.

Knowledge Of

- Marine law, regulations, and rules of the road;
- Basic principles involved with personnel and public relation practices;
- Principles and practices of modern lifesaving techniques, of small craft, harbor, and boating safety, and of equipment and apparatus used;
- Rules and regulations and applicable laws and ordinances;
- First aid practices and principles of specialized paramedical techniques;
- Basic law enforcement practices, dealing with the laws of arrest and search and seizure;
- Principles and practices of underwater search and recovery techniques and basic diving physics.

Ability To

- Supervise the activities of permanent and recurrent personnel;
- Supervise training program;
- Prepare clear, concise reports and review reports of subordinate personnel;
- Maintain outstanding public relations and service;
- Swim in adverse weather and surf conditions for extended periods of time;
- Maintain discipline and evaluate performances of subordinate personnel;

- Interpret and explain relative ordinances, regulations, rules of the road, and basic law enforcement practices dealing with the laws of arrest and search and seizure;
- Operate a high speed harbor patrol vessel under varying weather and surface conditions;
- Use compass, fathometer, and other navigational aids;
- Supervise and perform emergency underwater rescue and recovery operations with the use of self-contained breathing apparatus.

Marine Safety Boat Operator

Definition

Under supervision, operates a lifeguard rescue boat engaged in patrolling beach area, performs emergency lifesaving operations, and does related work as required.

Typical Tasks

The marine safety boat operator operates an ocean rescue vessel and supervises subordinate personnel assigned thereto; maintains daily records of engine performance and logs boat activities; makes periodical inspections of the boat's hull for dry rot, leaking seams, and cracks; periodically inspects boat's fittings and mechanisms, such as propellers, shafts, rudders, struts, fiber bearings, water intakes, ignition system, carburetors, generators, and so forth; supervises underwater dragging operations and installation of moorings; descends beneath the water surface for the recovery of bodies and the inspection of hulls and underwater fittings; operates a ship-to-shore radio and navigational instruments; performs routine boat maintenance operations such as painting, scraping, engine lubrication, and line repair; advises marine mechanics of defective and malfunctioning equipment; may personally engage in rescuing swimmers and in the administration of artificial respiration and other first aid techniques; may enforce laws relative to the use of public beaches and swimming areas; is capable of maintaining the operation of resuscitator, inhalator, and aspirator equipment; is subject to twenty-four-hour emergency call; is responsible for marine safety protection; and performs highly skilled operational tasks in rough weather and surf conditions.

Employment Standards

- High school graduate or G.E.D.;
- Two-years experience as an ocean lifeguard;
- Valid U.S. Coast Guard license for Class A Boat Operator;

- Valid first aid instructor's certificate issued by American Red Cross Association or emergency medical technician—1 rating;
- Certification from recognized police officer's academy;
- Minimum age, twenty-one years;
- Valid drivers license;
- Scuba certification from recognized authority;
- Cardio-pulmonary resuscitation instructor's certificate from recognized authority.

Knowledge Of

- Piloting and dead-reckoning navigation;
- Principles and practices of modern lifesaving techniques and of equipment used;
- First aid principles and practices including specialized paramedical techniques;
- Marine law, regulations, and rules of the road;
- Basic law enforcement practices dealing with the laws of arrest and search and seizure;
- Department rules and regulations and applicable laws and ordinances;
- Principles and practices of underwater search and recovery operations and basic diving physics;
- Basic hull design, repair, and marine engine maintenance.

Ability To

- Operate a high-speed powerboat under varying weather and ocean surface conditions;
- Operate directional finder, compass, and other navigational aids;
- Maintain discipline and supervise subordinate personnel;
- Prepare clear and concise reports;
- Size up emergency situations and adopt effective courses of action;
- Perform routine boat maintenance duties, including basic marine engine repairs;
- Swim in adverse weather and surf conditions and for extended periods of time;
- Perform emergency underwater rescue and recovery operations with the use of self-contained breathing apparatus.

Marine Safety Officer

Definition

Under supervision, patrols an assigned area in either an emergency rescue vehicle or patrol vessel in the first line protection of life, limb, and property; makes rescues; supervises recurrent personnel; and does related work as required.

Typical Tasks

The marine safety officer is responsible for marine safety protection; patrols assigned area in a radio-equipped mobile unit or patrol vessel, maintaining maximum security precautions and supervising recurrent personnel as needed; is constantly on the alert, making sure that all activity is in order; assumes charge in all rescue, first aid, and fire emergencies until relieved by superior officer; maintains and coordinates daily, weekly, and annual training programs for himself and his subordinate recurrent personnel; maintains discipline of the recurrent personnel under his supervision; supervises and participates in underwater rescue and recovery operations in his area; supervises first aid, lifesaving, and swimming drills; is responsible for maintaining all stations and vehicles in his area; writes clear and concise activity reports and funnels same to superior officer; enforces city ordinances and state harbor regulations and issues citations for same; makes periodic inspections of his vehicle or vessel and maintains daily records of engine performance and logs daily activities; performs underwater dragging operations and installs moorings and buoy markers; when assigned to patrol vessel, makes inspections of boat fitting and water intakes, ignition system, carburetors, and the like; removes hazardous objects from area; protects bathers and boaters and warns them of hazardous conditions; assists distressed vessels; is subject to twenty-four-hour emergency call; operates specialized lifesaving and fire-fighting equipment and performs various paramedical first aid practices of a highly skilled nature.

Employment Standards

- High school graduate or G.E.D., two years of college preferred;
- Two-seasons experience as ocean lifeguard;
- Successful completion of physical, oral, and written exam, including, but not limited to, mental aptitude, English, and grammar tests.
- Valid first aid instructor's certificate issued by the American Red Cross Association or emergency medical technician—1 rating;
- Minimum age, twenty-one years;
- Adequate hearing and visual activity;
- Valid drivers license;
- Scuba certification from recognized authority;
- Cardio-pulmonary resuscitation instructor's certification from recognized authority.

Knowledge Of

- Marine law, rules, and regulations, rules of the road;
- Piloting and dead-reckoning navigation;

- Rules and regulations of the department;
- Principles and practices of modern lifesaving techniques, of small craft harbor, and boating safety, and of equipment and apparatus used;
- First aid practices, including highly specialized paramedical techniques;
- Basic law enforcement practices dealing with the laws of arrest and search and seizure;
- Principles and practices of underwater search and recovery techniques and basic diving physics.

Ability To

- Use compass, fathometer, and other navigational aids;
- Perform routine boat maintenance, including basic marine engine and minor mechanical repairs;
- Operate a high-speed harbor patrol vessel under varying weather and water surface conditions;
- Size up emergencies and adopt effective courses of action;
- Prepare clear and concise reports;
- Maintain outstanding public relations and service;
- Swim in adverse weather and surf conditions for extended period of time;
- Maintain discipline and supervision of subordinate recurrent personnel;
- Perform underwater search and recovery operations;
- Maintain constant observation of an assigned area and note any signs of danger.

Lifeguard

Definition

Under supervision, guards an area of beach from an assigned station or, in some instances, patrols a section of beach in a mobile unit, in the protection of life, limb, and property; enforces beach regulations; makes rescues; and does related work as required.

Typical Tasks

The lifeguard watches designated section of beach and water from an assigned station or mobile unit; protects bathers and warns them of dangerous conditions; maintains telephone or radio communications with headquarters; rescues persons in distress or danger of drowning; answers inquiries and gives information pertaining to beaches; applies first aid to those in need, including highly specialized techniques such as mouth-to-mouth rescue breathing and heart-lung resuscitation; operates resuscitator, inhalator, and aspirator equipment; enforces beach regulations pertaining to safety and conduct; keeps logs on tides, weather and surf condition, rescues, first aid, and other miscellaneous services; turns in to his area supervisor clear, concise reports of daily activities; removes hazardous obstacles from sand and water; maintains a professional and courteous relationship with the public; and is responsible for marine safety protection.

Employment Standards

- Minimum age, sixteen years;
- Adequate hearing and visual activity;
- Excellent health;
- Valid advanced first aid card, issued by American Red Cross or emergency medical technician—1 rating;
- Successful completion of training program (minimum of fifty-six hours) and physical exam;
- Valid drivers license.

Knowledge Of

- All applicable rules and regulations;
- Principles and practices of livesaving techniques and equipment and apparatus used;
- First aid practices, including specialized paramedical techniques.

Ability To

- Maintain outstanding public relations and service;
- Swim in adverse weather and surf conditions for extended periods of time;
- Size up emergency situations and adopt effective courses of action;
- Maintain constant observation of area assigned, noting any signs of danger.

GENERAL POLICIES AND PROCEDURES

It is imperative to the success of any marine safety or lifeguard service, large or small, that written rules and regulations be established. Said regulations should be explicit and cover all phases of the lifeguard's responsibilities while on or off duty. In addition to those orders defining departmental policy and procedure relating to uniform specification, use and care of vehicles and equipment, special use and/or tactical laws, and boat operation, set standards governing the chain of command and the lifeguard's personal habits and behavior are a must. Following are excerpts from a General Order Manual utilized by several major services on the West Coast.

Suggested Regulations for Lifeguards

A. The chain of command from the administrative head on down in rank and line of authority shall be preserved. RANK SHALL NOT BE BYPASSED.

B. When in the presence of the public or other persons or employees of the service, officers shall be addressed by their official title.

C. The chief shall keep his commanding officers informed of changes within the command of order, assignment, and such where it concerns persons under their supervision. The commanding officer will similarly keep subordinate personnel informed, except in cases of emergency necessitating other action.

D. Any of the following violations shall result in disciplinary action.

    1. Drinking intoxicating liquor while on duty or reporting for duty with an obvious odor of liquor on breath or under the influence of any alcoholic beverage or drug.

    2. Conduct unbecoming an employee of the service.

    3. Insubordination.

    4. Immoral conduct.

    5. Neglect of duty.

    6. Conviction for violation of any criminal law.

    7. Inattention to duty.

    8. Sleeping while on duty.

    9. Laziness.

    10. Disorderly conduct.

    11. Disobedience of order.

    12. Leaving prescribed duties or area without authorization from supervisor or before being properly relieved.

    13. Being absent from duty without permission.

    14. Neglect to treat supervisor and members of the department and all other persons courteously and respectfully at all times.

    15. Willful maltreatment of the public (always address public as "sir" or "ma'am").

    16. Failure to direct to supervisors questions that employee cannot answer or does not have the authority to answer.

    17. Making false reports to the department, such as "sick or injured" for the purpose of obtaining time off.

    18. Neglecting to wear proper uniform or dress while on duty.

    19. Neglecting to maintain personal hygiene and good grooming.

    20. Gossiping about a fellow employee or employees concerning said employee's personal character or conduct to the detriment of any such employee.

    21. Receiving bribes in form of money, valuables, fees, rewards, or gifts of any kind from any person.

    22. Publicly criticizing the official action of a superior officer.

    23. Neglecting to report any member of the service known to be guilty of any violation of any rule, general order, or policy issued for the guidance of the service.

    24. Undue talking or visiting with employees or citizens, except while on official business, while on duty.

    25. Discussing official business of the service with others, both in and outside the service. When an employee is reprimanded by a

supervisor, or instructed, counseled, or corrected, said conference shall be held privately and exclusive of other employees. Following said conference, the subordinate shall not discuss the matter with other members of the department. No employee shall relieve another employee who is on duty without approval from his supervisor. Members must treat as confidential the official business of the service.

26. Loitering in any public place.
27. Failure to accept and follow requests and orders of immediate superior to the full extent of ability.
28. Failure to seek assistance from immediate supervisor for any problem employee cannot solve.
29. Failure to conduct self in a manner that will foster the greatest harmony and cooperation between mutual agencies and the general public.
30. Being late or failing to attend work or mandatory meeting without expressed consent from the immediate supervisor.
31. Failure to report for extra duty when so ordered.
32. Failure to maintain a soldierly bearing when on duty and to avoid a slovenly attitude of mind and body.
33. Taking to observational station reading matter, radio, musical instrument, or any other material that would distract attention from duty.
34. Failure to familiarize self with all details of operations and rules and regulations governing the service.
35. Refusing to accept "on call" status or extra duty when on days off or with advance notice, when on vacation.

Suggested Additional Rules for Ocean Lifeguards

1. Take all possible precautions to prevent accidents in the surf and on the beach and render efficient service to those in need.
2. Check beach area for riptides, holes, currents, or hazardous objects such as logs or glass at the start of a tour of duty.
3. Be responsible daily for knowing the water and air temperatures, high and low tides, and official hours of sunrise and sunset.
4. Maintain a physical fitness program that will enable adequate performance of all duties.
5. Enter into all conditions and training activities at the discretion of the supervisor.
6. Check all equipment at the start of tour of duty, making sure it is in adequate working condition.

Suggested Uniform Regulations

The importance of a professional looking and functional uniform cannot be overemphasized. Department morale and esprit de corps are greatly enhanced when the lifeguard wears a neat and good looking uniform, and a prestigious appearance will have a highly favorable effect on the public. A lifeguard's appearance will have a great effect on his attitude. A lifeguard whose uniform lends dignity and pride to his profession will tend to develop and display these same characteristics in the performance of his duty. Whenever possible, uniformity of dress should be maintained throughout the entire force.

General Philosophy

In selecting the proper uniform, the following should be considered

1. *Geographical Climate.* Material should be comfortable and of a weight conducive to prevailing temperatures. In areas where seasonal climates change radically, it is recommended that uniform specifications for both summer and winter be established.
2. *Quality.* Material of superior quality, while it may be more expensive, will insure a neat appearance and provide longer wear. Easily laundered fabrics are also desirable.
3. *Style.* In selecting a style, the prime concern should be the functionalism of the garment. It is imperative that the lifeguard uniform permit quick and easy movement and that foul weather apparel be designed in such a manner as to allow it to be shed quickly.
4. *Color.* Gaudy colors are not recommended nor are vivid, sharply contrasting colors. Conservative tans, browns, and navy blues are widely used by most organizations for their professional appearance and because they are less vulnerable to stains and soil marks.
5. *Identifying Insignia.* Some type of insignia, preferably a shoulder or breast patch, should be sewn on the uniform. Badges that denote authority along with additional items identifying rank are strongly recommended as they enhance the prestige of the uniform and represent a convenience to the public.

Specific Instructions

1. Lifeguards will at no time wear their uniforms or any identifying insignias when off duty.
2. Lifeguards shall wear the uniform prescribed for their particular assignment or station.
3. When the uniform is worn, care shall be taken to see that it fits well and is neat, clean, and properly pressed and that all metal goods are clean and shiny at all times.

SELECTION, RECRUITMENT, AND TRAINING

Because of the complexity and potential violence of the environmental conditions, as well as the number and range of client types handled in this environment, selection of personnel understandably requires some processes not applicable to other functions in the field of public safety. If a marine safety operation is going to be effective under today's tactical planning and execution methods, its lifeguards must be physically capable of handling many functions that a qualified police officer or fireman can do and also possess the ability to swim in heavy surf regardless of its violence for extended periods. He is not only swimming for himself, but is concerned with sustaining the safety of other individuals while he is working. Ocean lifeguards along coastal beaches are required to do this with strength and speed, which are often developed by the strenuous workout sessions of competitive water polo and swimming programs, from which guards are often recruited.

A trained ability to recognize and handle either impending or ongoing trouble of any description under any degree of environmental violence, when developed within an individual, is of special significance. A guard must be able to think out and plan how to handle the problem physically either acting alone or as a member of a team, or to function as a communications observer, assisting in the direction of an operation. Any decision he makes must be immediate and right. He will be faced with rapid fire decisionmaking repeatedly throughout his tour of duty.

The foregoing is not meant to imply that today's ocean lifeguard is the epitome of perfection. However, it does indicate the demands and stresses of lifeguarding. Therefore, an individual capable of meeting such demands is desirable for recruitment.

Selection

In selecting the best-qualified candidates for employment, no effort or expense should be spared. The training of a marine safety or lifeguard specialist is an expensive and lengthy process, especially in those services that incorporate underwater rescue operations and have law enforcement, paramedical, and/or fire suppression responsibilities. Training of an applicant who is unfit for the service may constitute a monetary loss in excess of the expenditure of the entire selection process, not to mention the loss of prestige that the department might suffer due to the poor judgement or misconduct of an individual not suited for the service.

Communities close to the ocean offer the best source of labor and have excellent high school and college programs in competitive water sports. Thus, a prospective employee's experience with surf, as well as his experience in the self-discipline needed to withstand the pain and rigors of training in these sports, will often give him a decided advantage in qualification tests. Invariably, success in qualifying is due to knowledge of ocean surf and currents, in addition to swimming and running capabilities and performance in front of an oral interview board. Another point in an applicant's favor is that usually he has embarked upon a self-training program to compete against other candidates, which requires strong self-discipline.

The modern-day lifeguard, faced with a rapidly changing society, may have to deal with a variety of complicated problems. Therefore, a good degree of intelligence is required. The working environment is both static and in violent motion, thus requiring repeated decisions and revisions throughout the day. Mass confusion, generated by both the environment and the public, will be his to unravel, and he must be able to immediately facilitate an orderly solution, either alone or as part of a team effort.

Guards handle lost children, crowd control, major and minor injuries, community relations, sex offenses, thefts of property, and almost all forms of client dissidence, including uses of narcotics or drunk and disorderly conduct. He is there when a problem first arises. How a situation develops after starting will depend upon his intelligence in handling it until support arrives—if it arrives.

The recruit's potential to handle such situations is evaluated in physical, written, and oral examination processes. These are administered by departmental staff groups that have had experience and have survived in this environment.

The individual who seems quietly and politely confident that he can get the task accomplished appeared best suited to lifeguarding. However, experience shows that a number of suitable personality types exist and do survive in extended employment, provided one common trait is retained. This is stability under stress, whether the issue is personal or in the line of duty.

Health, or measuring health alone, is here almost academic. Health is certainly a prerequisite, but physical conditioning is the critical criterion that separates successful candidates from the masses of "healthy," "fit" individuals unable to gain employment in an ocean lifeguard agency. Current competitive examination criteria have left the healthy per se individual behind.

Recruitment

Some agencies find that posting easily read examination announcements at local high schools, junior colleges, and universities will generally produce reasonably good results in attracting qualified candidates for recurrent or seasonal employment. Although this process attracts many who are physically unqualified, it is considered successful in view of the number of excellently conditioned individuals present when the examination begins.

Although generally unpublicized as an attraction process, the direct contact method is probably one of the most effective. When the department's employees actively seek to influence qualified candidates to join their ranks, it can produce excellent results. Currently successful employees will have outstanding judgement of an individual's capabilities to qualify. Usually, respect is one of the values judged.

As in the other public safety agencies, the seasonal ocean lifeguard selection processes are designed to eliminate unqualified candidates and to rank the remaining individuals in order of their qualification. However, there is difference in emphasis during the preliminary stages of testing, mainly in evaluating all the candidates' physical capabilities and conditioning while under "raw" competition in the working environment. Since running, swimming, and coping with heavy surf are the prerequisites, they must be judged before anything else.

Qualifying Examination

Use of a qualifying examination program allows the service to recruit the highest caliber of personnel available. Following is a recommended qualifying exam procedure that could be utilized in whole or in part by any marine safety or lifeguard service.

Physical Exam

1. 1000-meter ocean swim;
2. 400-meter ocean swim;
3. 1000-meter run–swim–run–swim–run.

Oral Interview

Prior to selecting candidates for a prehiring comprehensive training program, a brief oral board examination is often held in house in order to gain enough insight into the background and character of the applicant to enable the service to screen out those who are undesirable or who have a sub-par potential for learning.

The Training Program

If at all feasible, approximately twice the number of applicants in relation to job openings should be placed in the preservice training program. Invariably, through the course of the training session, some applicants will drop out of their own accord, and others will be eliminated by the instructional staff. It is also extremely advantageous to have an alternate hiring list of trained personnel, since openings may develop throughout the year, and the cost of additional training programs for one or two persons would be prohibitive.

The United States Lifesaving Association has developed the following training program curriculum for three basic lifeguard classifications. Each individual agency could of course adopt the classification that would best fit their needs. Said determination may also be affected by the financial capability of the governing body.

United States Lifesaving Association
Certification Requirements
Class III—Ocean Lifeguard

Training Program (minimum 24 hours—recommended 30 hours)
Orientation (6–8 hours)
1. Objectives and Goals of Program
2. Rules and Regulations
3. General Operating Procedures
4. Chain of Command
5. Environmental Hazards
   a. Riptides
   b. In-shore Holes
   c. Backwash
   d. Lateral Currents
   e. Other Geographical Abnormalities
   f. Dangerous Marine Life
6. Introduction to Equipment and Facilities
   a. Rescue Buoys
   b. Rescue Boards
   c. Boats and Vehicles
   d. Towers
   e. Other
7. Introduction to "Job of a Lifeguard"
   Skills Performed
   b. Responsibilities
   c. Physical Fitness
   d. Preventative Actions
   e. Public Relations
8. Communications
   a. Whistle and Hand Signals
   b. Other (i.e., radio, telephone)
9. Report Writing
Lifesaving Skills & Procedures (10–12 Hours)
1. Signs of Distress
2. Rescues with Equipment
   a. Basic Fundamentals
   b. General Types
   c. Compounded Rescues
   d. Rescue Variations

e. Skin and SCUBA Diving Rescues
3. Rescues Without Equipment
    a. Basic Fundamentals
    b. Technique Variations

Advanced First Aid (6–7 hours)
1. Severe Bleeding
2. Unconsciousness (cause unknown)
3. Heat Stroke and Heat Exhaustion
4. Burns
5. Care and Transportation of Spinal Injuries
6. Heart Attack
7. Alcohol and Drug Overdose
8. Fixation Splinting

Paramedical First Aid (2–3 hours)
(Certification from authorized agent recommended)
Cardio-Pulmonary Resuscitation

United States Lifesaving Association
Certification Requirements
Class II—Ocean Lifeguard

Training Program (minimum 32 hours—recommended 40 **hours**)
Orientation (8–10 hours)
1. Objectives and Goals of Program
2. General Orders—Rules and Regulations—Disciplinary **Policy**
3. Chain of Command and Scope of **Authority**
4. Environmental Hazards
    a. Riptides
    b. Backwash
    c. Inshore Holes
    d. Lateral Currents
    e. Piers, Groins, Jetties
    f. Dangerous Marine Life
5. Introduction to Equipment and Facilities
    a. Rescue Buoys
    b. Rescue Boards
    c. Vessels
    d. Vehicles
    e. Stations and/or Towers
    f. Binoculars
    g. Fins
    h. Other
6. Introduction to "Job of a Lifeguard"
    a. Skills Performed
    b. Responsibilities
    c. Physical Fitness and In-service **Training**
    d. Preventative Actions
    e. Public Relations
7. Communications
    a. Hand and Whistle Signals
    b. Telephone Procedures
    c. Radio Procedures

8. Report Writing
Lifesaving Skills & Procedures (14–16 hours)
1. Signs of Distress
2. Rescues with Equipment
   a. Basic Fundamentals
   b. Types of Rescues
   c. Compounded Rescues
   d. Rescue Variations
   e. Pier Rescues
   f. Boat Rescues
   g. Paddleboard Rescues
   h. Skin and SCUBA Diving Rescues
   i. Cliff Rescues
3. Rescues without Equipment
   a. Basic Fundamentals
   b. Technique Variations
Advanced First Aid (6–8 hours)
1. Severe Bleeding
2. Unconsciousness (cause unknown)
3. Heat Stroke and Heat Exhaustion
4. Care and Transportation of Spinal Injuries
5. Diabetes
6. Epilepsy
7. Heart Attacks and Strokes
8. Traction Splinting
9. Burns
10. Over-exposure to Cold
11. Skin and SCUBA Illnesses and Injuries
12. Alcohol and Drug Overdose

United States Lifesaving Association
Certification Requirements
Class I—Ocean Lifeguard

Training Program (minimum 56 hours)
Orientation (10 hours)
1. Objectives and Goals of Program
2. General Orders—Rules and Regulations—Disciplinary Policy
3. Chain of Command and Scope of Authority
4. Environmental Hazards
   a. Riptides
   b. Backwash
   c. Inshore Holes
   d. Lateral Currents
   e. Piers, Groins, Jetties
   f. Dangerous Marine Life
5. Introduction to Equipment and Facilities
   a. Rescue Buoys
   b. Rescue Boards
   c. Vessels
   d. Vehicles
   e. Stations and/or Towers

    f. Binoculars

    g. Fins

    h. Other

  6. Introduction to "Job of a Lifeguard"

    Skills Performed

    b. Responsibilities

    c. Physical Fitness and In-service Training

    d. Preventative Actions

    e. Public Relations

  7. Communications

    a. Hand and Whistle Signals

    b. Telephone Procedures

    c. Radio Procedures

  8. Report Writing

Lifesaving Skills and Procedures (20 hours)

  1. Signs of Distress

  2. Rescues with Equipment

    a. Basic Fundamentals

    b. Types of Rescues

    c. Compounded Rescues

    d. Rescue Variations

    e. Pier Rescues

    f. Boat Rescues

    g. Paddleboard Rescues

    h. Skin and SCUBA Diving Rescues

    i. Cliff Rescues

  3. Rescues without Equipment

    a. Basic Fundamentals

    b. Technique Variations

  4. Practical Applications

Emergency Care and Transportation of the Sick and Injured (15 hours)

  1. Severe Bleeding

  2. Unconsciousness (cause unknown)

  3. Heat Stroke and Heat Exhaustion

  4. Care and Transportation of Spinal Injuries

  5. Diabetes

  6. Epilepsy

  7. Heart Attacks and Strokes

  8. Traction Splinting

  9. Burns

  10. Over-exposure to Cold

  11. Skin and SCUBA Illnesses and Injuries

  12. Alcohol and Drug Overdose

  13. Cardio-Pulmonary Resuscitation

Practical and Written Examinations (11 hours)

  1. Written Exams on all Phases

  2. Practical Exams on all Phases

  3. Timed Swims

Performance Evaluation

Periodical performance evaluations of all personnel are also an extremely beneficial management tool. The performance of marine

PERFORMANCE RATING

EMPLOYEE_____CLASSIFICATION_____

Length of Time Under Your Supervision_____

CHARACTERISTICS	OUTSTANDING	ABOVE AVERAGE	AVERAGE	BELOW AVERAGE
General Attitude & Enthusiasm	_____	_____	_____	_____
Decisiveness/Self-Confidence	_____	_____	_____	_____
Dependability	_____	_____	_____	_____
Emotional Stability	_____	_____	_____	_____
Initiative	_____	_____	_____	_____
Compatability	_____	_____	_____	_____
Handles Public	_____	_____	_____	_____
Spots Rescues	_____	_____	_____	_____
Alertness	_____	_____	_____	_____
Performance in Emergencies	_____	_____	_____	_____
Punctuality	_____	_____	_____	_____
Requires Supervision	_____	_____	_____	_____
OVERALL PERFORMANCE	_____	_____	_____	_____

COMMENTS:_____
_____
_____
_____
_____
_____

Signature of Rating Officer_____

Date_____

PERFORMANCE EVALUATION REPORT

EMPLOYEE _____ DATE _____
POSITION _____ LAST REPORT DATE _____

Check items below as follows: + = Outstanding X = Above Average ✔ = Standard — = Weak	COMMENTS - STRENGTHS - WEAKNESSES - SUPERVISORY ABILITY

RATE EACH FACTOR:
Outstanding ———————————
Above Average ———————
Standard ———————
Weak ———

1. ATTITUDE: ☐☐☐☐ 1 2 3 4
    ☐ Toward dept. & its goals
    ☐ Desire to learn
    ☐ Self-confidence
    ☐ Self-development
    ☐ Willingness to participate
2. PERSONAL RELATIONS: ☐☐☐☐ 1 2 3 4
    ☐ Compatability
    ☐ Meeting & handling public
    ☐ Personal appearance
    ☐ Ability to express self
3. WORK HABITS: ☐☐☐☐ 1 2 3 4
    ☐ Punctuality
    ☐ Attendance
    ☐ Observance of rules & reg.
    ☐ Compliance with instruction
    ☐ Alertness & conscientiousness
    ☐ Application to duties
    ☐ Physical fitness
4. ABILITY: ☐☐☐☐ 1 2 3 4
    ☐ Leadership
    ☐ Spot rescues
    ☐ F.A. techniques
    ☐ Making decisions
    ☐ Work standards
5. ADAPTABILITY: ☐☐☐☐ 1 2 3 4
    ☐ Performance in emerg.
    ☐ Perf. with min. instr.
    ☐ Perf. in new situations
6. PRODUCTION: ☐☐☐☐ 1 2 3 4
    ☐ Rate of work
    ☐ Knowledge of job
    ☐ Compl. of work on schedule
7. QUALITY: ☐☐☐☐ 1 2 3 4
    ☐ Accuracy
    ☐ Written express.(rpt writing)
    ☐ Oral expression
    ☐ Neatness of work product
    ☐ Thoroughness

POINT TOTAL . . . . _____

Signatures of Reporting Officers	Over-all Evaluation			
	Weak	Standard	Above Aver.	Outstand.

RATER _____

REVIEWER _____ DATE _____

DEPT. HEAD _____ DATE _____

Report discussed with employee by:
                              DATE _____
This report has been discussed with me:
                              DATE _____

safety and lifeguard personnel must be periodically appraised for two primary reasons—(1) to discover those employees that are most qualified for promotions or special assignments; and (2) to detect deficiencies in the job performance that could be alleviated through improved recruitment procedures, training programs, or operating procedures.

There are two types of service-rating forms that a service might use. Form A should be prepared on a semiannual, quarterly, or monthly basis and serve as a spot check on an individual's progress in the interim period between the more detailed evaluation (Form B), which would be prepared on an annual basis. The evaluation of personnel by supervisors also stimulates their supervisory abilities and serves as a basis by which they themselves can be evaluated by their superiors.

MANAGEMENT PRACTICES

In addition to directing the activities of the organization, management personnel are also responsible for planning, research, and budgeting. In a small service these functions would be handled solely by the head administrator. In a larger service, however, several staff personnel would probably be involved in varying degrees.

Marine safety and lifeguard organizations who attempt to let their operations run by themselves on a day-to-day basis and rely on the ability of the operational personnel to cope with new problems and emergency situations as they arise will soon find themselves faced with a deteriorating organization flushed with chaotic confusion and a general lowering of morale throughout the ranks. Budget requests may fall by the wayside due to inadequate planning, and a substantial loss in departmental efficiency will be inevitable.

Planning and Research

In order for a marine safety service to stay abreast of current problems and insure their ability to cope with future needs, frequent reevaluation of equipment, facilities, personnel, and operational methods and procedures must be made. Although planning and research are the direct responsibility of management personnel, the entire working force should be involved as much as possible. The discovery of needs and supporting evidence thereof can originate from any level of authority and quite often does, especially in a larger organization employing several semi-independent divisions.

The recognition of a need is almost always the result of an efficient inspection program or in the field experience. The wise administrator will therefore be extremely attentive to the recommendations of subordinate personnel, expecially in a large organization where he is only indirectly involved with daily activities and must rely to a great extent on the ability of his staff to make responsible decisions.

Following the recognition of a need, a thorough research analysis should be conducted relative to what is presently being accomplished and what the total effect on the department will be when the change is instituted.

Budgeting

Efficient planning and research will further enable the chief administrator to adequately evaluate future money needs for personnel, equipment, and capital improvements. Such needs must be thoroughly justified in order to obtain the necessary appropriations, and therefore, surveys should be conducted to determine the need for replacing outdated and/or worn out equipment and meeting projected increases in demand by the public (i.e., towers, communications, rescue equipment, maintenance, and so forth). In simple terms, a budget is merely a work program based on the money needed to operate it successfully. Budgets should be justified on the theory that if the funds are not approved, some phase of service to the public will have to be either sacrificed or depleted to the point where it will become weak and vulnerable.

The appropriating authority must also be made fully aware that budget reduction in any critical areas will result in corresponding reductions in service to the public. The practice of "padding" the budget is not generally considered a desirable procedure since it tends to indicate a lack of confidence in and respect for the authorizing body and can be overcome through means of efficient planning, corroborating facts, figures, and substantiating criteria.

It should be pointed out that the legislative or governing body will determine the level of service it desires. However, it is the responsibility of the lifeguard administrative staff to thoroughly orientate said body with the scope of their service and the problems particular to their areas of responsibility to insure that the budget requests are evaluated objectively. It is a wise practice of the lifeguard administrator to submit annual reports to his governing body prior to budget time, outlining present operations and future goals. Said report should be supplemented with accurate facts and figures relative to departmental activities.

Marine Safety Glossary

ABAFT. Aft of, to the rear of.

ABEAM. On the side of the vessel, amidships or at right angles.

ABOUT. To go on the opposite tack, change directions.

ABYSS. A particularly deep part of the ocean, any part over 300 fathoms.

ACCRETION. Natural accretion is the gradual build-up of land over a long period solely due to the action of the forces of nature, on a beach by deposit of water-borne or airborne material. Artificial accretion is a similar build-up of land due to an act of man, such as the accretion formed by a groin, breakwater, or beach fill deposited by mechanical means.

ACORN BARNACLE. (rock barnacle). A barnacle whose shell is attached or cemented directly to a firm surface.

ADRIFT. Floating at the mercy of wind or current.

AFT. Toward the stern of the vessel.

AGROUND. Vessel touching bottom. Common names: grounded, on the beach, beached.

AIR EMBOLISM. Diving disease caused by excess air pressure within the lungs, resulting in a rupture of the air sacs, blood vessels, or the complete lung.

AMIDSHIPS. The middle point between bow and stern.

ANCHORAGE. An area where a vessel anchors or may anchor, either because of suitability or designation.

ANOXIA. (also anoxemia). The absence of oxygen, an abnormal condition produced by breathing air deficient in oxygen.

ANTIFOULING PAINT. (antifouling coat). A substance applied to a surface to prevent the attachment of marine organisms when submerged in water.

AQUALUNG. Underwater breathing apparatus. Cylinder containing compressed air, worn under water, from which to breathe. Common name: lung.

ARTIFICIAL RESUSCITATION. Resuscitation sequence done manually, without the aid of a machine.

ASH BREEZE. Absence of wind; calm.

ASPIRATOR. Tool used to clean or clear the air passages of an asphyxiated or nonbreathing patient, to clear such obstructions as body fluid or food regurgitation.

ASSIST RESCUE. Talk, swim, paddle, maneuver a boat, wade, run, climb, or descend to guide persons or property capable of making the safety of a beach, safe ground, or safe water on their own power, with or without partial physical contact. Common name: run, assist, preventative action.

ASTERN. Behind a vessel, in a backward direction, toward the stern.

AVERAGE DEPTH. The average water depths based on previous soundings.

AWASH. Tossed about or bathed by waves or tide.

BACKBOARD. A rigid flat board providing maximum immoblization used as a stretcher to transport a person suspected of having sustained a back or neck injury.

BACK RUSH. See Back Wash.

BACKUP. Lifeguard personnel or equipment called to an area to assist or stand by a rescue operation. Common name: rolling out unit, support, supplements, follow-up.

BACK WASH. Seaward return of water following the up rush of a wave on the beach. Seaward motion of water created by waves or chop striking an obstruction or steep incline on the beach. Common names: chop, undertow, surge.

BACKWATER. Water turned back by an obstruction, opposing current, or the like.

BALLAST. Broken stone, gravel, or other heavy material used in a vessel, usually a ship, to improve stability or control the draft.

BAR. A submerged or emerged embankment of sand, gravel, or mud built on the sea floor in shallow water by waves and currents.

BAROMETER. An instrument for measuring atmospheric pressure. Used also as a means of predicting changes in the weather.

BAR PORT. A harbor that can be entered only when the tide rises sufficiently to permit passage of vessels over a bar.

BASIN. A depression of the sea floor more or less equidimensional in form and of variable extent.

BATHER. Person who goes into the water for recreation but does not swim, usually walks, wades, stands in shallow water. Common names: fanny dipper, wader.

BATHYMETRIC CHART. A map delineating the form of the bottom of a body of water, usually by means of depth contours.

BEACH. The zone of unconsolidated material that extends landward from the low water line where there is marked changed in material or physiographic form or to the line of permanent vegetation.

BEACH BREAK. Waves breaking in long lines on a sloping sand beach.

BEACH EROSION. The carrying away of beach materials by wave action, tidal currents, littoral currents, or wind.

BEAM. The vessel's maximum width.

BEAM SEA. Wind at right angles to a vessel's keel.

BEARING. The direction of an object from an observer.

BECALM. A sailing vessel is becalmed when there is no wind. Common name: irons.

BELLY BOARD. A small surfboard or similar inflexible object ridden in a prone position. Common name: paipo board.

BENDS. Scuba-diving disease caused by too much nitrogen in the bloodstream from a saturation dive not following the decompression rules. Common name: compressed air illness, caisson disease.

BERM. A narrow shelf, path, or ledge created by wave action on the sand.

BILGE. Lower internal part of vessel's hull.

BILLOW. Usually a great wave or surge of water; any wave.

BITTS. Posts fitted into vessel's deck for securing mooring line.

BLIND ROLLERS. Long, high swells that have increased in height almost to the breaking point as they pass over shoals or run in shoaling water.

BLOWING SPRAY. Spray lifted from the sea surface by the wind and blown about in such quantities that the horizontal visibility is restricted.

BLOWN OUT. An undesirable surface condition caused by extreme winds rendering the surf unfavorable for aquatic activities.

BOARD SURFING. Any activity that involves riding waves with the use of a surfboard or being carried along or propelled by the action of waves with the use or aid of a surfboard. To board surf shall mean to do or engage in board surfing. Common names: surfing, riding.

BODY SKIMMING. Sliding along the beach on thin water in a prone position after gaining momentum from running and leaping forward. Common name: body whopping.

BODY SURFING. Riding a wave without the aid of a floating device. Common name: body whopping.

BOIL. Up-welling of water caused by a swell riding or striking shallow water or rock formations, causing a visual disturbance on the water surface. Common names: up-swelling, swirls.

BOSUN'S CHAIR. Seat by which a person in a sitting position can be lowered or elevated down or up the face of a cliff, embankment, building, pier, or the like.

BOTTOM CHARACTERISTICS. The type of material of which the bottom is composed and its physical characteristics, such as hard, sticky, rocky, kelp, sand, and so forth. Common name: bottom makeup.

BOTTOM FORMATION. Underwater structures.

BOTTOM SAMPLE. A portion of the material forming the bottom, brought up for inspection.

BOW. Forward part of a vessel.

BREAKER. A wave breaking on the shore, over shoal water or reef, a wave that has lots of sound as it spills over. Common name: crasher.

BREAKWATER. A structure protecting a shore area, harbor, anchorage, or basin from waves or current. Common names: seawall, jetties.

BRIM LINE. The edge around a body of water.

BROACH. To slip sideways in a wave or swell, veer or yaw dangerously.

BUDDY SYSTEM. Two persons, usually divers, working together in the water to obtain a common goal. Swimming, diving together for safety, each protecting the other from any danger.

BULKHEAD. Any upright partition separating compartments on a vessel, a wall or embankment for holding back earth.

BUOY LINE. A line supported by buoys, used to mark off a restricted water activity area, usually in a still water area.

CALM. The state or condition of the water surface when there is no wind, waves, or surface disturbances.

CAN RACK. Emergency storage rack for rescue buoys.

CAT'S PAW. A puff of wind; a light breeze affecting a small area, as one that causes patches of ripples on the surface of a water area.

CHAFE. To rub or damage by rubbing. Anything used to prevent it is called "chafing gear."

CHANNEL. (1) A natural or artificial waterway that periodically or continuously contains moving water or that forms a connecting link between two bodies of water. (2) The part of a body of water deep enough to be used for navigation through an area otherwise too shallow for navigation. The deepest portion of a stream, bay, or rip current through which the main volume or current of water flows.

CHOCK. A heavy casting of metal or wood with two short horn-shaped arms curving inward, between which ropes or hawser may pass for towing, mooring, and so forth.

CHOP. Disturbed surface of water usually caused by strong wind or after-effects of waves. Common name: white caps.

CLEAT. A fitting to which a line may be secured.

CLIFF RIG. An emergency vehicle equipped to answer any call to persons trapped below or on cliff faces.

CLOSE HAULED. Set of sail, roughly parallel length of vessel, when sailing in the direction of the wind. Common name: reefing.

COAST. The general region of indefinite width that extends from the sea inland to the first major change in terrain features.

COASTAL CURRENT. A relatively uniform drift usually flowing parallel to the shore in the deep water adjacent to the surf line. The current may be related to tides, winds, or distribution of mass. Common name: offshore current.

COMBER. A deep water wave whose crest is pushed forward by a strong wind and that is much larger than a white cap.

CONTROL ZONE. Area open to surfboarding on a temporary basis. Usually surfboarding is allowed at preset hours, eliminating all surfboards during peak swimming hours. Common name: aquatic control area.

CORAL. (1) The hard calcareous skeleton of various authrozoams and a few hydrozoams, the stony solidified mass number of such skeletons. In warm water colonial coral forms extensive reefs of limestone. In cool or cold water coral usually appears in the form of isolated solitary individuals. Occasionally, large reefs formed in cold waters by calcareous algae have been referred to as a coral. (2) The entire animal, a compound polyp, that produces the skeleton.

CORAL HEAD. A massive mushroom or pillar-shaped coral growth.

CORAL REEF. A ridge or mass of limestone built up of detrital material deposited around a framework of the skeletal remains of mollusks, colonial coral, and massive calcareous algae. Coral may constitute less than half of the reef material.

COUNTERCURRENT. A current flowing adjacent to the main current but in the opposite direction.

CRASHER. Wave breaking hard from top to bottom. Common names: pounder, coming over, heavy, sand buster, cruncher.

CREST. The highest part of a wave.

CREST WIDTH. The length of a wave along its crest.

CURL. The curved portion of a wave, which breaks progressively parallel in either direction while moving toward the beach.

CURRENT. The flowing of a stream of water at a greater velocity than that of the adjacent water. Common name: water movement.

CURRENT BASE. The maximum water depth below which currents are ineffective in moving sediment.

CURRENT DIRECTION. The direction toward which a current is flowing, called the set of the current. Example of a "south current" is a body of water flowing from north to south.

CURRENT PATTERN. The horizontal distribution of the surface or subsurface currents at various levels in a specified area.

DAILY INFORMATION BOARD. Sign displayed advising the public daily of weather and surf conditions, tides, temperatures, and size of surf.

DANGEROUS MARINE ANIMALS. Any water life that can inflict death, injury, or sickness to a person.

DAVIT. A form of crane for hoisting boats, anchors, cargo, and the like.

DEAD RECKONING. A method of navigation utilizing only the speed and heading of the craft, without reference to external aids.

DECOMPRESSION TABLES. Chart of rules to go by for saturation dives over thirty-three feet, using scuba gear. Common name: tables.

DEGREE. (1) A unit of temperature. (2) A unit of angular distance; $\frac{1}{360}$ part of a circle.

——. Indentation, hole, or break in surface of an object caused by water in motion striking that object against another object, rock, bottom, piling, or the like. Common name: perforate, crack, gouge, puncture.

DIVER'S FLAG. Square red flag with a white diagonal bar running across it from one corner to another. Warning especially to boats that divers are working in the area.

DOCUMENTED VESSEL. Vessel registered with the U. S. Bureau of Customs or the U. S. Coast Guard.

DORY. A hard chined, twenty-one-foot boat, usually rowed by two occupants or "dorymen" designed to be rowed in and through the surf zone. Common names: surf boat, bailer, and Cape Cod style.

DRAFT. The depth of water required to float a vessel.

DRAG. Parallel moving body of water in the surf zone usually moving away from the direction of the swell. Common names: long shore current, feeder.

DREDGE. A ship designed to remove sediment from a channel or bay to maintain draft depths.

DRIFT. Movement of water due to wave action, wind, or current.

DROP-OFF. Sudden increase in depth of water due to bottom formation. Common names: hole, shelf.

DROWNING. Asphyxiation by immersion in water or other liquid. Common name: deep six.

DRY SUIT. Thin waterproof rubber suit. Acts as an insulator when worn by a person in the water to retain body heat. Undergarments must be worn under the suit to aid in retaining the body heat. Common name: frogman suit.

EBB. The outgoing tide.

EBB CURRENT. The tidal current associated with the decrease in the height of a tide. Ebb currents generally set seaward or in the opposite direction to the tide progression. Erroneously called ebb tide. Common names: ebb tide, falling tide.

EDDY. A circular movement of water usually formed where currents pass obstructions, between two adjacent currents flowing counter to each other, or along the edge of a permanent current.

ELECTROLYSIS. Chemical decomposition of metals or alloys by the action of an electric current caused by contact with salt water.

EMBAYMENT. An indentation in a shore line forming an open bay.

EQUALIZING. Process of equalizing of all air spaces in the body, especially in the sinuses and ear canals, while submerging under water. Common name: clearing.

EQUATORIAL TIDES. Tides that occur approximately every two weeks when the moon is over the equator. At these times the moon produces minimum inequality between two successive high waters and two successive low waters.

EROSION. Any or all processes by which sand, soil, or rock is broken up and transported from one place to another.

ESTUARY. A tidal bay formed by submergence or drowning of the lower portion of a nonglaciated river valley and containing a measurable quantity of sea salt. Common names: drowned river mouth, branching bay, firth, frith.

FATHOM. Six-foot measure of ocean depth,

FATHOMETER. A machine to measure the depth of the water. Common names: depth gauge, depth finder, depth sounder.

FEATHERING. A wave just beginning to break, blowing white water on the peak of a wave caused by wind or momentum. Common names: knifer, hanging up.

FEEDER. Parallel-moving body of water that eventually will be turned seaward by a geological or manmade structure, forming a rip.

FEEDER CHANNELS. Channels parallel to shore along which feeder currents flow before converging to form the neck of a rip current.

FEELING BOTTOM. The action of a deep water wave on running into shoal water and beginning to be influenced by the bottom. Common name: peaks.

FENDERS. Cushions to protect a boat from bumping against a dock or another boat. Common name: bumpers.

FETCH. (1) An area of the sea surface over which seas are generated by a wind having constant direction and speed. (2) The length of the fetch area, measured in the direction of the wind in which the seas are generated. Common name: generating area.

FIRST AID. Immediate and temporary care given to a victim of an accident or sudden illness until the services of a doctor can be obtained.

FIRST AID ROOM. Part of Lifeguard facility set up to treat any type of water or beach injury or sickness. Area where injured or sick await transportation to hospital or home.

FLAG SYSTEM. Colored flags used to designate certain water activity zones or surf conditions.

FLOATING DEVICE. Any device that a person uses to support himself on the water surface. Common names: float, raft.

FLOOD. The incoming tide.

FLOTSAM. Floating debris, driftwood, and the like.

FLOW. The combination of tidal and nontidal current that represents the actual water movement.

FLOW NOISE. The noise produced by water moving past an object.

FOAM. Caused by air and water mixing, formed on the water's surface as waves break. Common names: soup, froth, white water.

FOAM LINE. The front of a wave as it advances shoreward after it has broken. Common names: soup line, white water.

FREE ASCENT. An emergency skill used in reaching the surface when the air supply is no longer available. Usually burdened gear is jettisoned before reaching the surface. Common names: bail out, ditching.

FREEBOARD. The vertical distance from the water to the gunwhale of a vessel.

FULLY DEVELOPED SEA. The maximum height to which ocean waves can be generated by a given wind force blowing over sufficient fetch, regardless of duration, as a result of all possible wave components in the spectrum being present with their maximum amount of spectral energy. Common name: fully arisen sea.

GANG GRAPNEL. A series of hooks set in a parallel pattern and used in the same fashion as a grappling hook.

GENERATION OF WAVES. (1) The creation of waves by natural or mechanical means. (2) The creation and growth of waves caused by a wind blowing over a water surface for a certain period of time.

GLASSY. Smooth, unrippled sea surface caused by absence of wind. Common names: glassed off, flat, lake.

GRAPPLING HOOK. An anchor with four, five, or more flukes or claws used to drag on the bottom to snag corpses or other objects. Used when water is too dirty to dive, usually a last resort.

GROIN. A breakwater extending at roughly right angles to the shore, usually designed to trap lateral drift and/or retard erosion of the shoreline. Common name: jetty.

GROUND SWELL. A long, high ocean swell.

GUARDED AREA. Water recreational area that has lifeguards on duty. Common names: guarded beach, covered area.

GUIDE LINES. Lines secured to an object to guide said object from injury. Lines attached to aid in control of a floating or suspended object.

GULLY. A relatively narrow ravine in the ocean bed.

GUNWHALE. The top of the hull side of a vessel. That part of a vessel where top sides and deck meet. Common name: rail.

GUTTER RIP. A short, powerful, fast-moving rip current found on a scalloped, steep, sloping beach front. These gutter rips often sweep people off their feet by surprise and into the next wave. The sweeping underwater current action is often confused with the term "undertow."

HARBOR. An area of water affording natural or manmade protection for vessels.

HAZE. The fine dust or salt particles dispersed through a portion of the atmosphere. The particles are so small that they cannot be felt or individually seen with the naked eye, but they diminish horizontal visibility and give the atmosphere a characteristic opalescent appearance that subdues all colors.

HEAD OF A RIP. Area where neck of rip disperses into the ocean body. Common names: rip head, dispersion area.

HEADQUARTERS. Lifeguard facility that houses the offices of the division's supervisors and administration. Has a public reception room, direct communication to all main towers, lifeguard boats, and vehicles. Usually has a workshop for maintenance and repairs, first air room, and storage for emergency vehicles and equipment. Is usually manned day and night all year.

HEAVY SEA. Severe water distrubance caused by winds or swell. Common name: rough sea.

HEAVY SURF. Large waves. Common names: heavies, surf's up, crashers, blue birds on the horizon.

HELM. Wheel or tiller by which a vessel is steered.

HELMSMAN. One who steers a vessel. Common names: driver, operator, pilot.

HIGH SIDING. Leaning body weight toward that side of a boat that is broadside and being pushed by a wave.

HIGH WATER LINE. The intersection of the plane of high water with the shore; it varies daily with the changing lunar phases and meteorological conditions. Common names: high water mark, beach line, tide line.

HURRICANE WAVE. A sudden rise in the level of the sea associated with a hurricane. Common names: hurricane surge, hurricane tide.

HYDROFOIL. A vessel equipped with planes that provide lift when the vessel is propelled forward.

HYPERVENTILATION. Excessive breathing in and out. Skindivers hyperventilate when preparing to hold their breath. Hyperventilation purges the breathing stimulant, carbon dioxide, out of the respiratory system and to a minor degree beefs up the percentage of oxygen in the lungs. Used incorrectly, it may cause unconsciousness. Common names: breathe deep, prepare to dive.

INHALATION. Allowing a patient to breathe at will air or oxygen administered by an apparatus. Common name: maintenance breathing.

INHALATOR. Machine used to administer a fresh flow of oxygen or air to a breathing patient at near or slight suffocation.

INLET. A short, narrow waterway connecting a bay or lagoon with the sea. When it is in its natural state, an inlet maintained by tidal currents, the name tidal inlet or tidal outlet is applied.

INSIDE. Term to indicate anything between the outside waves just beginning to break and the shoreline.

INTERSECTING WAVES. One of the component waves that, when superimposed on others, produces cross-swells. Common names: sugarloaf sea, pyramidal sea.

INTERTIDAL AREA. That portion of the shoreline lying between the high and low tide lines.

INVERSE ESTUARY. An estuary in which evaporation exceeds land drainage plus precipitation with resulting mixture of high salinity estuarine water and sea water.

INVERSION LAYER. A layer of water in which temperature increases with depth.

ISTHMUS. A narrow strip of land, bordered on both sides by water, that connects two larger bodies of land.

JETTISON. The throwing overboard of objects, especially to lighten a craft in distress. The taking off of articles from a person to allow more buoyancy, such as the weight belt from a skin diver.

JETTY. A breakwater extending into a body of water to prevent shoaling at the mouth of a river or entrance to a bay. Common name: breakwater.

JUNIOR GUARD. Young boy or girl volunteering free time in an organized group taught by professional lifeguards to learn lifeguarding techniques. Common names: nipper, J.G.

KEEL. A longitudinal structure extending along the center of the bottom of a vessel that gives main support to the vessel's hull bottom. It often projects below the bottom. Common names: center line, skag.

KELP. The general name for large species of seaweeds. Common names: weeds, seaweed, plant life.

KNEE BOARD. A type of belly board designed and used to surf in a kneeling position.

KNOT. One nautical mile per hour (nautical mile is 1.15 times a statute mile.)

LAGOON. A shallow sound, pond, or lake generally separated from the open ocean.

LANDLINE. Line swum out to a victim or victims caught in a rip and used to pull them back through the neck of the rip. Usually used as a last resort and on rock beaches. Common names: reel, line, lifeline.

LANDMARKS. A conspicuous object on land or sea that marks a locality or a visual line-up of two or more fixed objects on the beach to obtain a precise location on the water surface. Common name: marks.

LEAD LINE. A line, wire, or cord used in sounding.

LEEWARD. On side away from the wind.

LIFEGUARD BOAT. Vessel used by lifeguards to save lives and property, vessel used by lifeguards to patrol an assigned area. Common names: rescue boat, patrol boat, surf boat.

LIFEGUARD EQUIPMENT. Aids used by lifeguard in preventing accidents, death and bodily harm.

LIFEGUARD FACILITY. Building used to house lifeguard personnel and equipment. Common names: lifeguard station, lifeguard post.

LIFEGUARD STAND. Elevated observation post without first aid or storage facilities. Has direct communication to a main station. Usually manned only in the busy season. Common names: seasonal tower, bird cage, supplementary tower.

LIFEGUARD TOWER. Elevated observation used by lifeguard personnel to scan an assigned area. Common names: lifeguard stand, bird cage, tower, station, crow's nest.

LIFEGUARD VEHICLE. Vehicle used to transport backup lifeguards and lifesaving equipment to needed areas, vehicle used by lifeguards to patrol an assigned area. Common names: jeep, rescue vehicle, patrol jeep, dune buggy, four-wheel drive vehicle, mobile unit, area unit, lifeguard truck.

LITTORAL DRIFT. The material moved in the littoral zone under the influence of waves and currents.

LITTORAL TRANSPORT. The movement of material along the shore in the littoral zone by waves and currents.

LOG BOOK. Book kept at main stations, on rescue boats, and in emergency vehicles listing pertinent daily activities and times. Used as a reference for administration to justify needs.

LONG-CRESTED WAVE. A wave, the crest width of which is long compared to the wave length.

LOW WATER. The lowest limit of the surface water level reached by the lowering or outgoing tide.

LULL. Period of slack water between a set of waves. Common names: slack, periods.

LUNAR TIDE. That part of the tide caused solely by the tide-producing forces of the moon as distinguished from that part caused by the forces of the sun.

MAIN TOWER. A lifeguard station, usually manned all year, that supplies assistance to other lifeguard facilities in a given area. Common names: station zero, mother station, central vantage tower, control tower.

MAKATEA. The raised fin of a coral reef.

MAKE FAST. To belay or secure a rope.

MARKER BUOY. Any floating object secured to a line to the bottom, marking a location or submerged object. Common name: marker.

MARSH. An area of soft wet land. Flat land periodically flooded by salt water is called a "salt marsh." Common name: slough.

MARSH BAR. A narrow ridge of sand at the edge of a marsh undergoing wave attack.

MAT SURF. Surfing waves with the aid of an air-filled, semiflexible object. Common names: air mattress, rubber raft, float.

MEAN HIGH WATER. (MHW). The average height of all high waters recorded over a nineteen year period or a computed equivalent period.

MEAN LOW WATER. (MLW). The average height of all the low water recorded over a nineteen-year period or a computed equivalent period.

MECHANICAL RESUSCITATION. Resuscitation done with the aid of a machine. Common name: breathing device, resuscitator.

MIXED LAYER. The layer of the water that is mixed through wave action or thermohaline convection.

MOORING. An anchored buoy to which a boat secures when not in use. Common name: mooring buoy.

MOUTHPIECE. The breathing end of a snorkel or scuba suit.

MOUTH-TO-MOUTH. Resuscitation sequence where a rescuer blows air from his mouth into a nonbreathing victim's mouth, inflating the victim's lungs rhythmically, without the aid of a tube.

MUD FLAT. A muddy or sandy coastal strip usually submerged by high tide.

NARCOSIS. (nitrogen narcosis). A state of stupor or arrested activity, drunkenness caused by high pressure nitrogen from diving with compressed air at depths usually near or over 200 feet. Common name: rapture of the deep.

NEAR DROWNING. Person aided to the safety of a beach and administered resuscitation or inhalation who would have died by asphyxiation without this aid. Common name: close call.

NECK. Part of a rip where most drownings and rescues take place.

NONTIDAL CURRENT. Any current that is caused by other than tide-producing forces.

NOTICE TO MARINERS. A periodic publication containing information affecting the safety of navigation.

OBSERVER. Term used to describe a person in a vessel delegated to watch a person or object being towed by said vessel.

OCEAN CURRENT. A movement of ocean water characterized by regularity, either of a cyclic nature or more commonly as a continuous stream flowing along a definable path; a current not associated with wave action on the beach or water movement caused by changing tides in a narrow channel or bay entrance.

OFFSHORE WIND. A wind blowing seaward from the land in a coastal area. Common names: land breeze, opposing wind.

ONE-FEEDER RIP. Rip generated by one water supply source.

ONSHORE WIND. A wind blowing landward from the sea in a coastal area. Common name: sea breeze.

OPEN WATER. A relatively large area of free navigable water. Common name: open ocean.

OUTFLOW. The flow of water from the river or its estuary to the sea.

OUTSIDE. Used as a noun to indicate anything outside the normal surf-line. Common names: back side, out back.

OUTSIDE CALL. Any rescue call to an area not directly lifeguarded or an area not designated by an ordinance as a surfing zone, swimming area, control zone. Phone call received by a lifeguard communication center other than its own interdepartmental system. Common names: outside, outside line.

OVERFALLS. Breaking waves caused by opposing currents or by the wind moving against the current.

OVER THE FALLS. Object or person falling without control from wave peak to the wave bottom. Common names: wipeout, wiped out, down the tubes, lunched, creamed.

PAINTER. A short line attached to bow of a small boat.

PASSAGE. A narrow navigable pass or channel between two land masses or shoals.

PATROL. Walking or driving in an emergency vehicle, with ready rescue gear, in either a designated or a nondesignated area to investigate blind areas away from observation towers, to investigate a situation at closer range, or to communicate with persons in questionable situations. Common names: beach check, beach run, cruise.

PEAK. The top of a wave at the maximum point before breaking.

PEARL. The dipping of the bow of any floating object that has a designated forward part underwater at the base of any wave or swell, after gaining momentum from that swell or wave, causing that object to go out of control or submerge. Common names: nose in, wipe out.

PERMANENT LIFEGUARD. Person who is employed all year as a lifeguard and whose principal occupation is lifeguard. Common names: full-time guard, permanent man, year-round man.

PERMANENT SEASONAL GUARD. Lifeguard working under the title of part-time or seasonal guard, but working full time, usually filling a vacant permanent position on a temporary basis. Common names: permanent recurrent, long seasonal, permanent limited.

PLUNGE POINT. (1). For a plunging wave, the point at which the wave curls over and falls. (2). The final breaking point of the wave just before they rush up on the beach.

PLUNGING WAVE. Wave that tends to curl over and breaks with a crash. Common names: crasher, heavy, lot of water, breaker.

POD. A number of sea animals closely clustered together on the ocean surface, such as seals, whales, and so forth. Common name: school.

POLLUTED WATER. The impairment of the quality of water by chemical or thermal wastes. Common names: dirty, scum water.

POOR STROKE. Description of a swimmer with poor swimming style, a person who is getting no power out of his swimming style. Common names: tourist, flat lander, thrasher, inlander.

PORT. Side of vessel to left when facing forward.

POSTED AREA. Area that has signs, flags, or signals regulating water and beach activities. Designated area, signed area.

POT HOLE. A hole in the ocean floor in the surf line a few feet or yards in diameter. Common names: hole, inshore hole.

PREVAILING CURRENT. The flow most frequently observed during a given period, usually a month, season, or year. Common name: prevailing drag.

QUICK RELEASE. Buckle or snap that can be pulled open by one hand, releasing a load or burden.

RACE. A very fast current flowing through a relatively narrow channel.

RADIO CODE. A number of words abbreviating messages to eliminate lengthy radio conversations. Method used to keep radio clear for emergencies. Common names: code list, codes, code.

READY ABOUT. Order given to stand by to tack sailing ship.

RECOMPRESSION. The treatment of decompression sickness or air embolism in a recompression chamber using the treatment tables.

RED TIDE. Rust-colored water in the day that causes the white water to glow at night and caused by dinoflagellate plankton bloom, usually in the spring and summer. Common names: plankton, luminous, dynoflangate.

REEF. Any hard geographical structure that is underwater at high tide. Common names: rock, rock structure, coral head.

REEF BREAK. Isolated waves breaking over shallow waters of a reef. Common name: peak bread.

REFLECTED WAVE. A wave that is returned seaward when it impinges upon a very steep beach, barrier, or other reflecting surface. Common name: back wash.

REFRACTION OF WATER WAVES. (1) The process by which the direction of a wave in shallow water at an angle to the contours is changed. That part of the wave advancing in shallower water moves more slowly than the other part still advancing in deeper water, causing the wave crest to bend toward alignment with the underwater contours. (2) The bending of wave crests by currents.

REGULATOR. An automatic mechanical device for maintaining or adjusting the high pressure flow of air from an aqualung tank to the external water pressure, allowing a diver to breathe underwater at any depth.

REPETITIVE DIVE. More than one saturation dive over thirty-three feet using scuba gear. Common name: repeat.

RESCUE. To swim, paddle, maneuver a boat, wade, run, climb, or descend to render aid to persons or property in distress. To bring or deliver persons or property from any confinement or danger. To regain or recover. Common names: run, save, pull out.

RESCUE BOARD. Usually a large surfboard over ten feet long, over twenty-five inches wide, and over three and a half inches thick. Used to make long-range rescues in mild surf and to apprehend surfboard violators. Common names: lifeguard board, paddle board.

RESCUE BOAT. Powerboat, usually twin screw, used outside and sometimes inside surfline to assist the beach lifeguard in the protection of swimmers, surfboarders, and boatmen. Used in harbors and bays. Lifeguard rescue boats do not undertake U.S. Coast Guard functions but do answer sea disaster calls upon Coast Guard request. Common names: patrol boat, lifeguard boat.

RESCUE BUOY. Cylinder flotation device secured by a line to a shoulder sling, harness, or belt worn by a lifeguard to effect a swimming rescue or an assist. Common names: torpedo buoy, can rescue tube, can buoy.

RESTING STROKE. Swimming stroke used to rest the body but not to lose progress in a current. Momentary change of swimming style. A swimming style not as powerful as could be exerted. Common names: sidestroke, breaststroke.

RESURGENCE. The continued rising and falling of a bay or semienclosed water body many hours after the passage of a severe storm.

RESUSCITATION. Process of rhythmically inflating the lungs of an asphyxiated patient with air or oxygen in an attempt to maintain life.

RESUSCITATOR. Machine used to rhythmically inflate the lungs of an asphyxiated victim with oxygen or atmosphere air.

RETARDATION. The amount of time by which corresponding tidal phases grow later day by day (averages approximately fifty minutes).

RILL MARK. A small groove, furrow, or channel made in mud or sand on a beach by tiny streams following an outflowing tide.

RIP CURRENT. Body of water traveling seaward generated by wave action or tide. Common names: rip, riptide, sea puss, hole, seaward current.

RIPPLE. The ruffling of the surface of water, hence a little curling wave or undulation.

ROCK BEACH. Any beach that has rock structures extending into the water.

ROLLER. An indefinite term used to describe one of a series of waves, usually a long-crested wave that rolls up a beach, large breaker on an exposed coast formed by a swell coming from a great distance.

RUDDER. The device used for steering and maneuvering a boat.

RUN. Lifeguard or equipment on route to a rescue or assist. Assist or rescue in progress. Common names: rescue, assist, emergency, Code 3, response.

RUN-UP. The rush of water up a structure on the breaking of a wave. The amount of run-up is the vertial height above still water level that the rush of water reaches.

SAFETY HELMET. Head gear worn to protect the head from injury. Common names: helmet, hat, surfing helmet.

SAND BAR. Island of sand submerged or exposed in the surfline. Common names: bar, shoal.

SAND CHANNEL. Sand area underwater or exposed at low tide, surrounded by reefs, rocks, or kelp. Common name: sand spit.

SCUBA. Self-contained underwater breathing apparatus, any breathing unit that is free of surface functions taken underwater by a diver.

SCULL. An oar used at the stern of a boat to propel it forward with a thwartwise motion.

SEA ANCHOR. An anchor not reaching the botton that acts in the way a parachute does.

SEABOARD. A general term for the rather extensive coastal region bordering the sea.

SEA BREEZE. A light wind blowing toward the land caused by unequal heating of land and water masses.

SEA CAVE. A cave eroded in a sea cliff by wave action. It usually is at sea level. Common name: marine cave.

SEA CLIFF. A cliff situated at the seaward edge of a coast.

SEA LEVEL. The height of the surface of the sea at any level. Common name: water level.

SEARCH PATTERN. Preset pattern used by personnel in locating person or objects on the surface or submerged. Common name: search line.

SEASHORE LAKE. A body of water isolated from the sea by sediment bars or banks.

SEASONAL CURRENT. A current that changes with seasonal winds.

SEASONAL LIFEGUARD. Lifeguard employed during the summer months, vacations, weekends and holidays, usually an hourly employee. Common names: recurrent guard, weekend guard, part-time guard, guard as needed, temporary guard, summer guard.

SEA STACK. A tall, columnar rock isolated from the coast by differential wave erosion.

SEA WALL. A manmade structure of rock or concrete built along a portion of coast to prevent wave erosion of the beach.

SEAWARD. In the direction of the sea.

SEAWEED. Any macroscopic marine algae or seagrass.

SEDIMENT. Any natural material carried in suspension by water. Causes underwater visibility obstruction. Common name: garbage.

SENIOR GUARD. A lifeguard who by virtue of experience, knowledge, and/or maturity has been assigned to a key station, tower, area, or special departmental function that carries with it added responsibility.

SET. Series of waves.

SHALLOWS. An indefinite term applied to expanses of shoal or shallow water.

SHALLOW WATER. Commonly, water of such a depth that surface waves are noticeably affected by bottom topography.

SHALLOW WATER BLACKOUT. Skin diver passing out underwater from the lack of oxygen or an unblance of carbon dioxide. Common name: blackout.

SHELF. A rock ledge, reef, or sandbank in the sea.

SHOAL. A submerged ridge, bank, or bar consisting of or covered by unconsolidated sediments (mud, sand, gravel) that is at or near enough to the water surface to constitute a danger to navigation. If composed of rock or coral, it is called a reef.

SHOALING. A bottom effect that describes the height of waves, but not the direction. It can be divided into two parts that occur simultaneously. In one part, waves become less dispersive close to shore, and since the same energy can be carried by high waves or those of lesser height, this effect causes a gradual decrease in the wave height. In the other part, the crests move closer together, and since the energy between crests remains relatively fixed, the waves can become higher near shore. These effects are seen in the initial decrease in height of the incoming wave, followed by an increase in height as the wave comes into shore.

SHOALING EFFECT. The alteration of a wave proceeding from deep water into shallow water.

SHORE BREAK. Waves peaking and breaking where the beach meets the water's edge. Common names: inside break, insiders.

SHORE FACE. The narrow zone seaward from the low tide shoreline permanently covered by water, over which the beach sands and gravels actively oscillate with changing wave conditions.

SHORE-CRESTED WAVE. A wave the crest length of which is of the same order of magnitude as the wave length. A system of short-crested waves has the appearance of hills being separated by troughs.

SIDE CURRENT. Body of water traveling parallel to shore generated by wave action, wind, or tide. Common names: drag, parallel drag, feeder, trough, lateral drift, long shore current.

SKEG. The afterpart of the keel of a vessel near the sternpost. The underneath aft fin of a surfboard or similar object used to prevent slippage and aid control of a surfboard or similar object when it is in motion. Common name: keel.

SKIM BOARD. A flat, thin board, usually round, ridden after being thrown into very shallow water over a flat sand beach.

SKIN DIVING. Submerging underwater from the surface without the use of scuba gear. Common name: free dive.

SKY GENIE. Trademark name used for a descending device that is operated by friction, used on cliff rescues.

SLACK WATER. The interval when the speed of the tidal current is very weak or zero; usually refers to the period of reversal between ebb and flood currents. Common name: slack tide.

SLIDER. Wave breaking with its white water sliding in an even motion down its face. Common name: feathering wave.

SMALL CRAFT WARNING. Storm signal warning pleasure craft vessels of dangerous water surface conditions caused by strong wind.

SNORKEL. A J-shaped tube held in the mouth that permits breathing when a person's face is just at water level or just under the surface.

SNUB. Check a rope suddenly. Common names: make fast, secure.

SOLAR TIDE. The tide caused solely by the tide-producing forces of the sun.

SOLITARY WAVE. A wave consisting of a single elevation, its height not necessarily small compared to the depth, and neither followed nor preceded by another elevation or depression of the wave surface.

SOUNDING. The measurement of the depth of water beneath a ship.

SPILLING WAVE. Wave breaking gradually over a considerable distance. Common name: slider.

SPORTS DIVER. One who submerges underwater, with or without scuba, for recreational purposes.

SPOUTING HORN. Marine cave eroded in coastal rocks that has top opening through which water spouts or sprays as waves surge into the cavern beneath. Common name: blow hole.

STAKE LINE. Heavy rope line used on cliff rescues that is hung over a cliff, most often supported by two or more stakes driven into the earth.

STAND BY. A state of readiness in which a lifeguard maintains a fixed location in preparation for a possible emergency response.

STAND OFF. To maintain surveillance directly in front of or adjacent to a possible rescue or other dangerous water situation.

STARBOARD. Side of vessel to right when facing forward.

STERN. After end of a vessel. Common name: transom.

STILL WATER. Body of water not having wave action, usually a bay or lake. Common names: flat water, calm water, glassed off, smooth.

STOKES BASKET. A contour stretcher constructed of tubular frame woven with wire mesh. Common names: litter, litter basket, basket, Stokes stretcher.

STORM SURF. Distorted waves, irregular wind-blown waves. Common names: slop, churned up, wind waves.

STORM SURGE. A rise above normal water level on the open coast due only to the action wind stress on the water surface. A storm surge is more severe when it occurs in conjunction with a high tide.

STRETCHER. Portable platform or body contour platform used to transport an injured or deceased person in a lying position. Common names: gurney, litter.

SUBTIDAL AREA. The area immediately below the low tide zone.

SUCKED UNDER. Object or person pulled under momentarily by churning water. Common names: wipeout, back door, lunched, clobbered, boiled.

SUMMER SEASON. That time of the year when public schools are out for summer vacation and lifeguard services are fully staffed with seasonal help. Common names: busy season, summer vacation.

SURF (noun). The swell of the sea that breaks upon the shore or shallow water causing white water. Common names: waves, breakers.

SURF (verb). To be propelled or gain momentum using the forward motion of a swell or wave with or without the aid of a floating device.

SURFACE DIVE. Submerging underwater from the water surface on own power. Common name: porpoising.

SURFACE WAVE. A progressive gravity wave in which the disturbance is confined to the upper limits of a body of water.

SURFBOARD. Any rigid, inflexible device upon which or with the use or aid of which a person can ride waves or be carried along or propelled by the action of waves. Common names: board, stick, gun.

SURF HAZARDS. Unsafe areas or conditions in the surf line.

SURFING. Riding or being propelled by the action of a wave with the aid of a surfboard. Common names: board surf, surfboarding.

SURFING AREA. Area open to surfboarding only, no swimming unless incidental to surfboarding.

SURF LINE. That area in which waves break, bordered on the outside by the most offshore break and on the inside by the most shoreward break.

SURF ZONE. Area between the furthest outside waves that are just beginning to break and the edge of the water on the beach. Common names: breaker line, surf zone, breaker zone.

SURF'S DOWN. Waves breaking smaller than normal. No surf at all. Common names: flattened out, flat, a lake.

SURF'S UP. Waves breaking larger than normal.

SURGE. A swelling or sweeping rush of water, a violent rising and falling of water. Common names: movement, boil.

SURGING WAVE. Wave that peaks up, but instead of spilling or plunging, slides up on the beach face.

SWASH. (1) The rush of water up onto the beach following a breaking wave. (2) A bar over which the sea washes. Common name: surge.

SWASH MARK. The thin wavy line of fine sand, mica scales, bits of seaweed, and the like left by the up-rush when it recedes from its upward limit of movement on the beach face. Common names: high water line, tide mark, tide line.

SWELL. Visual bump on the ocean surface that moves in one or several directions. Eventually forms a wave when striking shallow water.

SWIM FINS. Flat, webbed rubber footwear worn by swimmers to gain power and speed out of their kick. Common names: fins, flippers.

SWIMMING AREA. Water area open to swimming only.

THERMOCLINE. Temperature variation underwater; colder, denser water that is under a warmer water layer.

THOUGH. Parallel inshore channel in the ocean floor running a few to many yards in length. Common names: hole, feeder, trench, drop-off, channel.

THWARTS. A seat that runs across the beam of a boat or vessel. May or may not strengthen the hull.

TIDAL CURRENT. The alternating horizontal movement of water associated with the rise and fall of the tide caused by the astronomical tide-producing forces. In relatively open locations, the direction of tidal currents rotates continuously through 360 degrees diurnally or semi-diurnally. In coastal regions, the nature of tidal currents will be determined by local topography as well. Common names: tidal stream, tidal movement.

TIDAL DELTA. Sand bars or shoals formed in the entrance of inlets by reversing tidal currents.

TIDAL FLAT. A marsh or sandy or muddy coastal flatland that is covered and uncovered by the rise and fall of the tide. Common name: mud flat.

TIDAL WAVE. A great exchange of water caused by a strong force, usually from an earthquake centered in or near the ocean. The effect is a violent, sudden, extreme tide exchange on the beach resulting in probable damage to inlets, harbors, bays, ocean frontage, and so forth. Common names: tsunami, seismic wave.

TIDE. The periodic rising and falling of water with an accompanying horizontal movement resulting from the gravitational attraction of the moon and sun acting upon the rotating earth.

TIDELAND. Land that is under water at high tide and uncovered at low tide.

TIDE MARK. (1) A high water mark left by tidal water. (2) The highest point reached by a high tide. (3) A visual mark indicating any specified state of tide.

TIDE POOL. A pool of water remaining in the intertidal area after recession of the tide.

TIDE RACE. A very rapid tidal current in a narrow channel or passage.

—— The difference in height between consecutive high and low water.

TIDE TABLES. Tables that give daily predictions, usually a year in advance, of the times and heights of the tide. These predictions are usually supplemented by tidal differences and constants, by means of which additional predictions can be obtained for numerous other places.

TIDEWAY. A channel through which a tidal current flows.

TILLER. Bar or handle for turning a vessel's rudder.

TOPSIDE. Above the deck of a vessel. Common name: above deck.

TRANSVERSE BARS. Slightly submerged sand ridges that extend at right angles to the shoreline.

TRAVEL TIME. The time necessary for waves to travel a given distance from the generating area.

TREADING WATER. Maintaining stationary position on the surface of the water by using the legs and arms.

TSUNAMI. A sea wave produced by a submarine earthquake or volcanic, eruption. It may travel unnoticed across the ocean for thousands of miles from its point of origin and builds up to great heights over shoal water. Common names: tunami, tidal wave, seismic sea wave.

TWIRLY BENDS. Caused by trapped expanding air in the ear canal upon ascending. Can cause dizziness and nausea. In severe cases, the ear drum may perforate. Expanding air is trapped by mucus. Common names: sinus squeeze, reverse block.

TWO-FEEDER RIP. Rip generated by two water supply sources.

UNDA. The part of the ocean floor that lies in the zone of wave action, in which the bottom sediments are repeatedly stirred and reworked. The topographic expression is termed "undaform," and the rock unit is termed "undathem."

UNDERTOW. (1) A seaward flow near the bottom of a steep, sloping beach. (2) The subsurface return flow of the water carried up on shore by waves.

UNDERWAY. Vessel in motion, technically a vessel is underway when not moored, at anchor, or aground. Common name: moving.

UP COAST. In U. S. usage, the coastal direction trending toward the north.

UPLIFTED REEF. A coral reef exposed above the water.

UP-RUSH. The rush of water up onto the beach following the breaking of a wave.

UP-WELLING. Bottom water reaching the surface because of disturbance caused by swells, waves, or current. Up-welled water is usually cooler. Common name: boil.

VICTIM. Any person directly involved in an accident, incident, or rescue.

WAKE. Path of disturbed water left behind a moving vessel or moving object in the water.

WARNING. Verbal contact by voice or electronic equipment explaining an existing danger. To verbally move a person or crowd from a danger. Any verbal message on present beach safety conveyed to a daily attendance.

WATER ABILITY. Personal performance and endurance in all types of water conditions, such as surfing, diving, swimming, paddling, and so forth.

WATERSPOUT. Usually, a tornado occurring over water; rarely, a lesser whirlwind over water, comparable in intensity to a dust devil over land. Waterspouts are most common over tropical and subtropical water.

WAVE. (1) A disturbance that moves through or over the surface of the medium (here the ocean) with speed dependent upon the properties of the medium. (2) A ridge, deformation, or undulation of the surface of a liquid.

WAVE BASE. The depth at which wave action ceases to stir the sediments.

WAVE CREST. The highest part of a wave. Also that part of a wave above still water level.

WAVE FORECASTING. The theoretical determination of future wave characteristics, usually from observed or predicted meteorological phenomena.

WAVE FRONT. The leading side of a wave.

WAVE GENERATION. The creation of waves by natural or mechanical means. The growth of waves caused by a wind blowing over a water surface for certain periods of time. The area involved is called a "fetch."

WAVE TRAIN. A series of waves moving in the same direction. Common names: series, set.

WAVE TROUGH. The lowest part of a wave form between successive wave crests. Area between two ocean swells.

WAY. Movement of a vessel through the water.

WEIGHT BELT. Weight belt worn by a diver to compensate for buoyancy.

WET SUIT. Foam neoprene rubber suit that fits snugly to the body, worn by a person in the water to retain body heat. Water is allowed to enter the suit and is trapped and warmed by the body. Undergarments are not necessary under the suit. Common name: frogman suit.

WHITE CAP. Wind-blown chop that has white froth or foam appearance.

WHITE WATER. In the surf zone, water that is mixed with air causing it to turn white. Common names: soup, surge, slop, fizz, foam.

WIND-DRIVEN CURRENT. A current formed by the force of a wind.

WIND MIXING. Mechanical stirring of water due to motion induced by the surface wind.

WINDWARD. Into the wind, side wind is hitting. The direction from which the wind is blowing.

WIND WAVE. A wave resulting from the action of wind on a water surface. While wind is acting on it, it is called a sea; thereafter, a swell.

WINTER SEASON. The time of the year when schools are in session and beach attendance is at a minimum.

WIRED. To have superior knowledge and ability. Example: he has this surfing area "wired."

Index

251